Phacoemulsification in Difficult and Challenging Cases

Phacoemulsification in Difficult and Challenging Cases

Edited by

Luis W. Lu, M.D.
Clinical Instructor of Ophthalmology
University of Pittsburgh School of Medicine
St. Marys, Pennsylvania

I. Howard Fine, M.D.
Clinical Associate Professor of Ophthalmology
Oregon Health Sciences University
Eugene, Oregon

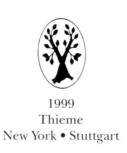

1999
Thieme
New York • Stuttgart

Thieme New York
333 Seventh Avenue
New York, NY 10001

Phacoemulsification in Difficult and Challenging Cases
Luis W. Lu, M.D.
I. Howard Fine, M.D.

Phacoemulsification in difficult and challenging cases / edited by
   Luis W. Lu and I. Howard Fine.
      p.   cm.
   Includes bibliographical references and index.
   ISBN 0-86577-791-8. — ISBN 3-13-114671-0
   1. Phacoemulsification.   I. Lu, Luis W. II.   Fine, I. Howard,
1936-
   [DNLM: 1. Phacoemulsification—methods.   2. Eye Diseases—surgery.
WW 260 P5315 1998]
RE451.P466 1999
617.7'42059—dc21
DNLM/DLC
for Library of Congress   98-4055
                                                                      CIP

Copyright © 1999 by Thieme Medical Publishers, Inc. This book, including all parts thereof, is legally protected by copyright. Any use, exploitation or commercialization outside the narrow limits set by copyright legislation, without the publisher's consent, is illegal and liable to prosecution. This applies in particular to photostat reproduction, copying, mimeographing or duplication of any kind, translating, preparation of microfilms, and electronic data processing and storage.

Important note: Medical knowledge is ever-changing. As new research and clinical experience broaden our knowledge, changes in treatment and drug therapy may be required. The authors and editors of the material herein have consulted sources believed to be reliable in their efforts to provide information that is complete and in accord with the standards accepted at the time of publication. However, in view of the possibility of human error by the authors, editors, or publisher of the work herein, or changes in medical knowledge, neither the authors, editors, publisher, nor any other party who has been involved in the preparation of this work, warrants that the information contained herein is in every respect accurate or complete, and they are not responsible for any errors or omissions or for the results obtained from use of such information. Readers are encouraged to confirm the information contained herein with other sources. For example, readers are advised to check the product information sheet included in the package of each drug they plan to administer to be certain that the information contained in this publication is accurate and that changes have not been made in the recommended dose or in the contraindications for administration. This recommendation is of particular importance in connection with new or infrequently used drugs.

Some of the product names, patents, and registered designs referred to in this book are in fact registered trademarks or proprietary names even though specific reference to this fact is not always made in the text. Therefore, the appearance of a name without designation as proprietary is not to be construed as a representation by the publisher that it is in the public domain.
Compositor: Compset. Printer: Götz
Printed in Germany
5 4 3 2 1
TNY ISBN 0-86577-791-8
GTV ISBN 3-13-114671-0

To my wonderful wife and best friend Laura, and to my sons L. Michael and Andrew for their loving understanding and support.

Luis W. Lu

My profound thanks to Vicky Fine, my lovely wife, through whose help and encouragement my career has developed in a spectacular way.

I. Howard Fine

Contents

Contributors		ix
Preface		xiii
Acknowledgments		xv

1. Phacoemulsification in Patients with Previous Keratorefractive Surgery — 1
   Jack T. Holladay and Wagner Zacharias
2. Phacoemulsification in Patients with High Myopia — 13
   Paul S. Koch
3. Phacoemulsification in High Hyperopic Cataract Patients — 21
   James P. Gills and Myra Cherchio
4. Phacoemulsification in Patients with High Astigmatism — 33
   Luis W. Lu and Stephen Hollis
5. Phacoemulsification in Patients with Fuchs' Corneal Dystrophy — 41
   Gavin G. Bahadur, Jack M. Dodick, and Richard P. Gibralter
6. Intraocular Lens Power Calculation in Triple Procedures — 49
   Olivia N. Serdarevic
7. Management of the Small Pupil in Phacoemulsification — 55
   Virgilio Centurión, I. Howard Fine, and Luis W. Lu
8. Phacoemulsification in Patients with Uveitis — 65
   Jorge L. Alío y Sanz and Enrique Chipont
9. Phacoemulsification in a Previous Functioning Glaucoma Surgery — 75
   Luis W. Lu
10. Phacoemulsification in Combined Cataract and Glaucoma Surgery — 83
    Alan S. Crandall
11. Phacoemulsification in Pseudoexfoliation — 91
    I. Howard Fine and Richard S. Hoffman
12. Phacoemulsification in Subluxated Cataracts — 99
    Andres Corét, Jorge Villar-Kuri, Yoshihiro Tokuda, and Luis W. Lu
13. Phacoemulsification in Intumescent and Rock Hard Cataracts — 111
    Abhay R. Vasavada, Jose A. Claros, and Raminder Singh

14	**Phacoemulsification in Posterior Polar Developmental Cataracts** *Abhay R. Vasavada and Raminder Singh*	121
15	**Phacoemulsification in Pediatric Patients** *Albert W. Biglan*	129
16	**Phacoemulsification Following Vitreoretinal Surgery** *Louis D. Nichamin*	145
17	**Phacoemulsification in Ocular Trauma** *Miguel Ângelo Padilha*	151
18	**Phacoemulsification in Severe Chronic Obstructive Pulmonary Disease** *I. Howard Fine and Richard S. Hoffman*	157
19	**Phacoemulsification in Patients with Bleeding Disorders** *Horacio U. Rotman, John Belardo, Ana C. Sanseau, and Luis W. Lu*	161
20	**Phacoemulsification in the Presence of Neovascularization of the Iris** *Ehud I. Assia*	169
21	**Phacoemulsification in Patients with High Risk of Choroidal Hemorrhage** *Guillermo A. Pereira and Luis W. Lu*	173
	Index	177

Contributors

Jorge L. Alío y Sanz, M.D.
Professor and Chairman
Department of Ophthalmology
University of Alicante School of Medicine
Director, Institutio Oftalmologico
 de Alicante
Alicante, Spain

Ehud I. Assia, M.D.
Chairman
Department of Ophthalmology
Meir Hospital
Sapir Medical Center
Kfar-Saba, Israel

Gavin G. Bahadur, M.D.
Fellow
Cornea and External Diseases
Department of Opthalmology
Manhattan Eye, Ear & Throat Hospital
New York, New York

John Belardo, M.D.
Director
Western Oklahoma Eye Center
Elk City, Oklahoma

Albert W. Biglan, M.D., F.A.C.S.
Adjunct Associate Professor
Department of Ophthalmology
University of Pittsburgh School of Medicine
Director
Pediatric Ophthalmology
Children's Hospital of Pittsburgh
Pittsburgh, Pennsylvania

Virgilio Centurión, M.D.
ISRS Representative for Latin America
Brazilian Society of Cataract and Refractive
 Surgery
Brazilian Society of Eye Banks
São Paulo, Brazil

Myra Cherchio, C.O.M.T.
Research Assistant
St. Luke's Cataract and Laser Institute
Tarpon Springs, Florida

Enrique Chipont, M.D.
Professor
Department of Ophthalmology
University of Alicante School of Medicine
Alicante, Spain

Jose A. Claros, M.D.
Staff Surgeon
Department of Ophthalmology
Hospital Conde De Valenciana
Mexico City, Mexico
Director
Instituto de Enfermedades y Cirugía Ocular
Mérida, Mexico

Andres Corét, M.D.
Director
Instituto Oftalmológico de Barcelona
Clinica Carmelitana
Autonomous University of Barcelona
Barcelona, Spain

Contributors

Alan S. Crandall, M.D.
Clinical Professor
Department of Ophthalmology
University of Utah Medical Center
Salt Lake City, Utah

Jack M. Dodick, M.D.
Chairman
Department of Ophthalmology
Manhattan Eye, Ear & Throat Hospital
Associate Clinical Professor of
  Ophthalmology
College of Physicians and Surgeons of
  Columbia University
New York, New York

I. Howard Fine, M.D.
Clinical Associate Professor
Department of Ophthalmology
Oregon Health Sciences University
Adjunct Professor of Health Education
University of Oregon
Eugene, Oregon

Richard P. Gibralter, M.D.
Director
Ophthalmology Residency Training
Director
Cornea Fellowship
Department of Ophthalmology
Manhattan Eye, Ear & Throat Hospital
New York, New York

James P. Gills, M.D.
Clinical Professor
Department of Ophthalmology
University of South Florida
Director
St. Luke's Cataract and Laser Institute
Tarpon Springs, Florida

Richard S. Hoffman, M.D.
Staff Surgeon
Oregon Eye Associates
Eugene, Oregon

Jack T. Holladay, M.D., F.A.C.S.
McNeese Professor
Department of Ophthalmology
University of Texas Medical School
  at Houston
Houston, Texas

Stephen Hollis, M.D.
Director
Hollis Eye Care Center
Columbus, Georgia

Paul S. Koch, M.D.
Director
Koch Eye Associates
Warwick, Rhode Island

Luis W. Lu, M.D.
Clinical Instructor
Department of Ophthalmology
University of Pittsburgh School of Medicine
Pittsburgh, Pennsylvania
Chief of Service
St. Marys Regional Medical Center
Elk County Regional Medical Center
Director
Elk County Eye Clinic
St. Marys, Pennsylvania

Louis D. Nichamin, M.D.
Director
Staff Surgeon
Laurel Eye Clinic
Brookville, Pennsylvania

Miguel Ângelo Padilha, M.D.
Professor
Department of Ophthalmology
UNI-Rio, Gama Filho University
President
Brazilian Society Ophthalmology
President
Latin-American Society of Cataract and
  Anterior Segment Surgeons
Rio de Janeiro, Brazil

Guillermo A. Pereira, M.D.
Director
Unidad Oftalmologica de Caracas
Associacion Venezolana Para El Avance De La
  Oftalmologia
Caracas, Venezuela

Horacio U. Rotman, M.D.
Professor
Universidad Nacional de Buenos Aires
Unidad Hospitalaria, Hospital Penna
Instituto De La Vision
Buenos Aires, Argentina

Ana C. Sanseau, M.D.
Staff Surgeon
Instituto De La Vision
Buenos Aires, Argentina

Olivia N. Serdarevic, M.D.
Director
Cornea Service
New York Hospital-Cornell University Medical Center
Assistant Professor of Clinical Ophthalmology
Department of Ophthalmology
Cornell University Medical College
Professeur D'Ophtalmologie
Universite De Paris
Paris, France

Raminder Singh, M.D.
Junior Consultant
Iladevi Cataract and IOL Research Centre
Raghudeep Eye Clinic
Memnagar, Ahmedabad
India

Yoshihiro Tokuda, M.D.
Chief Supervisor
Department of Ophthalmic Surgery
Inouye Eye Hospital
Tokyo, Japan

Abhay R. Vasavada, M.D.
Honorary Professor
Department of Ophthalmology
Gujarat University
Ahmedabad, India
Head
Iladevi Cataract and IOL Research Centre
Raghudeep Eye Clinic
Memnagar, Ahmedabad
India

Jorge Villar-Kuri, M.D.
Director
San Jose Institute
Post-Graduate Professor
Hospital Para Evitar La Ceguera En Mexico
Mexico City, Mexico

Wagner Zacharias, M.D.
Chief
Department of Ophthalmology
Hospital Brigadeiro
Chief,
Department of Ultrasonography
Instituto Tadeu Cvintal
São Paulo, Brazil

Preface

At the present time, phacoemulsification has achieved overwhelming dominance as the cataract extraction technique of choice in the United States.[1] It is spreading rapidly to all countries throughout the world, where it is increasingly utilized because of its inherent safety and its ability to achieve rapid visual rehabilitation and highly desirable refractive results. Cataract surgery by phacoemulsification allows a cure to take place at the time of the surgery without necessitating additional facilities and personnel to administer long and laborious postoperative care.

As surgeons become increasingly skilled in the variety of phacoemulsification techniques, they are getting results, which are very satisfying to themselves as well as their patients. All surgeons, however, are occasionally confronted with difficult and challenging cases, which might necessitate some deviation from the usual technique. The incidence of these cases is relatively small, but in each instance the surgeon is confronted with an unfamiliar challenge and is once again returned to the status of a relative newcomer to the procedure.

It is for this reason that this book was compiled. Because the authors are experts with sufficient skill and experience in each and every one of the difficult and challenging cases presented, phacoemulsification surgeons should find this book extremely useful prior to undertaking a difficult or unusual case. Although it is not viewed as a book that will be read from cover to cover during sequential sittings, it is certainly a book that will be referred to with great frequency as surgeons confront the difficult, unusual, or challenging case.

Each of the authors is highly experienced, a dedicated teacher, and a master of the technology. Their willingness to share their experiences and insights will be of benefit to those patients who are at unusual risk.

Luis W. Lu, M.D.
I. Howard Fine, M.D.

Reference
1. Learning DV. Practice styles and preferences of ASCRS members — 1996 survey. J Cat Refract Surg 1997;12:527–535.

Acknowledgments

We would like to recognize the following individuals for their valuable assistance in bringing this book into fruition: We thank Dr. Gary Torbey and Dr. Ricardo Galue who gave many hours perusing through the manuscript and offered valuable suggestions for improvement. We also extend our appreciation to Andrea Seils, Senior Medical Editor, Jinnie Kim, Editorial Assistant, and Pam Ritzer, Production Editor, of Thieme, for their tireless dedication to seeing this book through. Needless to say, their help was instrumental in the making of this book. We must also acknowledge the important contribution of so many leading experts in ophthalmology who authored the chapters in the book. There would not be a book without their willingness to share their experience and knowledge.

L.W.L.
I.H.F.

1

Phacoemulsification in Patients with Previous Keratorefractive Surgery

JACK T. HOLLADAY AND WAGNER ZACHARIAS

Several measurements of the eye are helpful in determining the appropriate intraocular lens power to achieve a desired refraction. These measurements include central corneal refractive power (k-readings), axial length (biometry), horizontal corneal diameter (horizontal white to white), anterior chamber depth, and lens thickness. The accuracy of predicting the necessary power of an intraocular lens is directly related to the accuracy of these measurements.[1,2]

Fyodorov first estimated the optical power of an intraocular lens using vergence formulas in 1967.[3] Between 1972 and 1975, when accurate ultrasonic A-scan units became commercially available, several investigators derived and published the theoretical vergence formula.[4-9] All of these formulas were identical[10] except for the form in which they were written and the choice of various constants such as retinal thickness, optical plane of the cornea, and optical plane of the intraocular lens. These slightly different constants accounted for less than 0.50 diopters in the predicted refraction. The variation in these constants was a result of differences in lens styles, A-scan units, keratometers, and surgical techniques among the investigators.

■ Primary Cataract Surgery. IOL Calculations Requiring Axial Length

Theoretical Formulas

The theoretical formula for intraocular lens power calculations has not changed in almost 30 years, since the original description by Fyodorov in 1967.[3] Although several investigators have presented the theoretical formula in different forms, there are no significant differences except for slight variations in the choice of retinal thickness and corneal index of refraction. There are six variables in the formula: (1) corneal power (K); (2) axial length (AL); (3) intraocular lens (IOL) power; (4) effective lens position (ELP); (5) desired refraction (DPostRx); and (6) vertex distance (V). Normally, the intraocular lens power is chosen as the dependent variable and solved for using the other five variables, where distances are given in millimeters and refractive powers given in diopters:

$$IOL = \frac{1336}{AL - ELP} - \frac{1336}{\frac{1336}{\frac{1000}{1000} + K} - ELP}$$

The only variable that cannot be chosen or measured preoperatively is the effective lens position (ELP). The improvements in intraocular lens power calculations over the past 30 years are a result of improving the predictability of the variable ELP. The term "effective lens position" (ELP) was adopted by the FDA in 1995 to describe the position of the lens in the eye, since the term anterior chamber depth (ACD) is not anatomically accurate for lenses in the posterior chamber and can lead to confusion for the clinician. The ELP for intraocular lenses before 1980 was a constant of 4 mm for every lens in every patient (first generation theoretical formula). This value actually worked well in most patients because the majority of lenses implanted were iris clip fixation, in which the principal plane averages approximately 4 mm posterior to the corneal vertex. In 1981, Binkhorst improved the prediction of ELP by using a single variable predictor, the axial length, as a scaling factor for ELP (second generation theoretical formula).[11] If the patient's axial length was 10% greater than normal (23.45 mm), he would increase the ELP by 10%. The average value of ELP was increased to 4.5 mm because the preferred location of an implant was in the ciliary sulcus, approximately 0.5 mm deeper than the iris plane. Also, most lenses were convex-plano, similar to the shape of the iris supported lenses. The average ELP in 1996 has increased to 5.25 mm. This increased distance has occurred primarily for two reasons: the majority of implanted IOLs are biconvex, moving the principal plane of the lens even deeper into the eye, and the desired location for the lens is in the capsular bag, which is 0.25 mm deeper than the ciliary sulcus.

In 1988, we proved[2] that using a two variable predictor, axial length and keratometry, could significantly improve the prediction of ELP, particularly in unusual eyes (third generation theoretical formula). The original Holladay 1 Formula was based on the geometrical relationships of the anterior segment. Although several investigators have modified the original Holladay 1, a two variable prediction formula, no comprehensive studies have shown any significant improvement using only these two variables.

In 1995, Olsen published a four variable predictor that used axial length, keratometry, preoperative anterior chamber depth, and lens thickness.[12] His results did show improvement over the current two variable prediction formulas. The explanation is very simple. The more information we have about the anterior segment, the better we can predict the ELP. This explanation is a well known theorem in prediction theory where the more variables that can be measured describing an event, the more precisely one can predict the outcome.

In a recent study,[13] we discovered that the anterior segment and posterior segment of the human eye are often not proportional in size, causing significant error in the prediction of the ELP in extremely short eyes (<20 mm). We found that even in eyes shorter than 20 mm, the anterior segment was completely normal in the majority of cases. Because the axial lengths were so short, the two variable prediction formulas severely underestimated the ELP, explaining part of the large hyperopic prediction errors with current two variable prediction formulas. After recognizing this problem, we began to take additional measurements on extremely short and extremely long eyes to determine if the prediction of ELP could be improved by knowing more about the anterior segment. Table 1–1 shows the clinical conditions that illustrate the independence of the anterior segment and the axial length.

Since 1996, we have been gathering data from 35 investigators around the world. Several additional measurements of the eye have been taken, but only seven preoperative variables (axial length, corneal power, horizontal corneal diameter, anterior chamber depth, lens thickness, preoperative refraction, and age) have been found to be useful for significantly improving the prediction of ELP in eyes ranging from 15 to 35 mm.

TABLE 1–1. Clinical Conditions Demonstrating the Independence of the Anterior Segment and Axial Length

Anterior Segment Size	Axial Length		
	Short	Normal	Long
Small	Small eye Nanopthalmos	Microcornea	Microcornea +Axial myopia
Normal	Axial hyperopia	Normal	Axial myopia
Large	Megalocornea Axial hyperopia	Megalocornea	Large Eye Buphthalmos +Axial myopia

The improved prediction of ELP is not totally due to the formula, but is also a function of the technical skills of the surgeons who are consistently implanting the lenses in the capsular bag. A 20.0 D IOL that is 0.5 mm axially displaced from the predicted ELP will result in approximately a 1.0 D error in the stabilized postoperative refraction. However, when using piggy-back lenses totaling 60.0 D, the same axial displacement of 0.5 mm will cause a 3.0 D refractive surprise; the error is directly proportional to the implanted lens power. This direct relationship to the lens power is why the problem is much less evident in extremely long eyes, since the implanted IOL is either low plus or minus to achieve emmetropia following cataract extraction.

The Holladay 2 Formula and the interim results of the 35 investigators were presented at the June 1996 ASCRS meeting in Seattle, Washington.[23] A-scan manufacturers and software programs have implemented the new formula since 1997.

Once these additional measurements become routine among clinicians, a new flurry of prediction formulas using seven or more variables will emerge, similar to the activity following our two variable prediction formula in 1988.[2] The standard of care will reach a new level of prediction accuracy for extremely unusual eyes, just as it has for normal eyes. Calculations on patients with axial lengths between 22 and 25 mm with corneal powers between 42.0 and 46.0 D will do well with current third generation formulas (Holladay 1[2], SRK/T[14] and Hoffer Q[15]). In cases outside this range, the Holladay 2 formula should be used to assure accuracy.

Piggy-Back IOLs to Achieve Powers Above 34 D

Patients with axial lengths shorter than 21 mm should be calculated using the Holladay 2 Formula. In these cases, the size of the anterior segment has been shown to be unrelated to the axial length.[13] In many of these cases, the anterior segment size is normal and only the posterior segment is abnormally short. In a few cases, however, the anterior segment is proportionately small to the axial length (nanophthalmos). The differences in the size of the anterior segment in these cases can cause an average of 5.0 D hyperopic error with third generation formulas because they predict the depth of the anterior chamber to be very shallow. Using the newer formula can reduce the prediction error in these eyes to less than 1.0 D.

Accurate measurements of axial length and corneal power are especially important in these cases because any error is magnified by the extreme dioptric powers of the IOLs. Placement of both lenses in the bag with the haptics aligned is essential. Inadvertently placing one lens in the bag and the other in the sulcus can cause a 4.0 D refractive surprise.

Determining the Corneal Power in Patients with Previous Keratorefractive Surgery (RK, PRK, and LASIK)

The number of patients who have had keratorefractive surgery (radial keratotomy (RK), photorefractive keratectomy (PRK), or laser-assisted in-situ keratomileusis (LASIK)) has been steadily increasing over the past 20 years. With the advent of the excimer laser, these numbers are predicted to increase dramatically. Determining their corneal power accurately is difficult and usually is the determining factor in the accuracy of the predicted refraction following cataract surgery. Providing this group of patients the same accuracy with intraocular lens power calculations as we have provided our standard cataract patients presents an especially difficult challenge for the clinician.

Methods of Determining Corneal Power

Accurately determining the central corneal refractive power is the most important and difficult part of the entire intraocular lens calculation process. The explanation is quite simple. Our current instruments for measuring corneal power make too many incorrect assumptions with corneas that have irregular astigmatism. The cornea can no longer be compared to a sphere centrally, the posterior radius of the cornea is no longer 1.2 mm steeper than the anterior corneal radius, etc. Because of these limitations, the calculated method and the trial hard contact lens method are most accurate, followed by corneal topography, automated keratometry, and finally manual keratometry.

Calculation Method

For the calculation method, three parameters must be known: the K-readings and refraction before the keratorefractive procedure and the stabilized refraction after the keratorefractive procedure. It is important that the stabilized postoperative refraction be measured before any myopic shifts from nuclear sclerotic cataracts occur. It is also possible for posterior subcapsular cataracts to cause an apparent myopic shift, similar to capsular opacification, where the patient wants more minus in the refraction to make the letters appear smaller and darker. The concept which we described in 1989 subtracts the change in refraction due to the keratorefractive procedure at the corneal plane from the original K-readings before the procedure, to arrive at a calculated postoperative K-reading.[16] This method is usually the most accurate because the preoperative Ks and refraction are usually accurate to ± 0.25 D. An example calculation to illustrate the calculation method is given.

Example:

Mean Preoperative K = 42.50 @ 90° and 41.50 @ 180° = 42.00 D
Preoperative Refraction = −10.00 + 1.00 × 90°, Vertex = 14 mm
Postoperative Refraction = −0.25 + 1.00 × 90°, Vertex = 14 mm

Step 1. Calculate the spheroequivalent refraction for refractions at the corneal plane (SEQ_C) from the spheroequivalent refractions at the spectacle plane (SEQ_S) at a given vertex, where

a. $SEQ = Sphere + 0.5\,(Cylinder)$

b. $SEQ_C = \dfrac{1000}{\dfrac{1000}{SEQ_S} - Vertex\,(mm)}$

Calculation for *preoperative* spheroequivalent refraction at corneal plane

a. $SEQ_R = -10.00 + 0.5 * (1.00) = -9.50\,D$

b. $SEQ_C = \dfrac{1000}{\dfrac{1000}{-9.50} - 14} = -8.38\,D$

Calculation for *postoperative* spheroequivalent refraction at corneal plane

a. $SEQ_R = -0.25 + 0.5 * (1.00) = +0.25\,D$

b. $SEQ_C = \dfrac{1000}{\dfrac{1000}{-0.25} - 14} = +0.25\,D$

Step 2. Calculate the change in refraction at the corneal plane.

Change in refraction = Preoperative SEQ_C − Postoperative SEQ_C
Change in refraction = −8.38 − (+0.025) = −8.68 D

Step 3. Determine calculated postoperative corneal refractive power.

Mean Postoperative K = Mean Preoperative K − Change in refraction at corneal plane
Mean Postoperative K = 42.00 − 8.68 = 33.32 D

This value is the calculated central power of the cornea following the keratorefractive procedure. For IOL programs requiring two K-readings, this value would be entered twice.

Trial Hard Contact Lens Method

The trial hard contact lens method requires a plano hard contact lens with a known base curve and a patient whose cataract does not prevent them from being refracted to approximately ± 0.50 D. This tolerance usually requires a visual acuity of better than 20/80. The patient's spheroequivalent refraction is determined by normal refraction. The refraction is then repeated with the hard contact lens in place. If the spheroequivalent refraction does not change with the contact lens, then the patient's cornea must have the same power as the base curve of the plano contact lens. If the patient has a *myopic shift* in the refraction with the contact lens, then the base curve of the contact lens is *stronger* than the cornea by the amount of the shift. If there is a *hyperopic shift* in the refraction with the contact lens, then the base curve of the contact lens is *weaker* than the cornea by the amount of the shift.

Example:

The patient has a current spheroequivalent refraction of +0.25 D. With a plano hard contact lens with a base curve of 35.00 D placed on the cornea, the spherical refraction changes to -2.00 D. Since the patient had a myopic shift with the contact lens, the cornea must be weaker than the base curve of the contact by 2.25 D. Therefore, the cornea must be 32.75 D (35.00 -2.25), which is slightly different than the value obtained by the calculation method. In equation form, we have

SEQ Refraction *without* hard
　　　contact lens = +0.25 D
Base Curve of Plano hard contact lens = 35.00 D
SEQ Refraction *with* hard contact lens =
　　　-2.00 D
Change in Refraction = $-2.00 - (+0.25)$
　　　= -2.25 D (myopic shift)
Mean Corneal Power = Base Curve of
　　　Plano HCL
　　　+ Change in Refraction
Mean Corneal Power = 35.00 + -2.25
　　　Mean Corneal Power = 32.75 D

N.B.—This method is limited by the accuracy of the refractions which may be limited by the cataract.

Corneal Topography

Current corneal topography units measure more than 5000 points over the entire cornea and more than 1000 points within the central 3 mm. This additional information provides greater accuracy in determining the power of corneas with irregular astigmatism compared to keratometers. The computer in topography units allows the measurement to account for the Stiles-Crawford effect, actual pupil size, etc. These algorithms allow a very accurate determination of the *anterior* surface of the cornea. However, they provide no information about the posterior surface of the cornea. In order to accurately determine the total power of the cornea, the power of both surfaces must be known.

In normal corneas that have not undergone keratorefractive surgery, the posterior radius of curvature of the cornea averages 1.2 mm less than the anterior surface.[17] In a person with an anterior corneal radius of 7.5 mm using the Standardized Keratometric Index of Refraction of 1.3375, the corneal power would be 45.00 D. Several studies have shown that this power overestimates the total power of the cornea by approximately 0.56 D. Hence, most IOL calculations today use a net index of refraction of 1.3333 (4/3) and the anterior radius of the cornea to calculate the net power of the cornea. Using this lower value, the total power of a cornea with an anterior radius of 7.5 mm would be 44.44 D. This index of refraction has provided excellent results in normal corneas for IOL calculations.

Following keratorefractive surgery, the assumptions that the central cornea can be approximated by a sphere (no significant irregular astigmatism or asphericity), and that the posterior corneal radius of curvature is 1.2 mm less than the anterior radius, are no longer true. Corneal topography instruments can account for the changes in the anterior surface, but are unable to account for any differences in the relationship to the posterior radius of curvature. In RK, the mechanism of having a peripheral bulge and central flattening apparently causes similar changes in both the anterior and posterior radius of curvature so that using the net index of refraction for the cornea (4/3) usually gives fairly accurate results, particularly for optical zones larger than 4 to 5 mm. In RKs with optical zones of 3 mm or less, the accuracy of the predicted corneal power diminishes. Whether this inaccuracy is due to the additional central irregularity with small optical zones or the difference in the relationship between the front and back radius of the cornea is unknown at this time. Studies measuring the posterior radius of the cornea in these patients will be necessary to answer this question.

In PRK and LASIK, the inaccuracies of these instruments to measure the net corneal power is almost entirely due to the change in the relationship of the radii of the front and back of the cornea, since the irregular astigmatism in the central 3 mm zone is usually minimal. In these two procedures, the anterior surface of the cornea is flattened with little or no effect on the posterior radius. Using a net index of refraction (4/3) will overestimate the power of the cornea by 14% of the change induced by the PRK or LASIK, that is, if patient had a 7 D change in the refraction at the corneal plane from a PRK or LASIK with spherical preoperative Ks of 44 D, the actual power of the cornea is 37 D and the topography units will give 38 D. If a 14 D change in the refraction has occurred at the corneal plane, the topography units will overestimate the power of the cornea by 2.0 D.

In summary, the corneal topography units do not provide accurate central corneal power following PRK, LASIK, and in RKs with optical zones of 3 mm or less. In RKs with larger optical zones the topography units become more reliable. The calculation method and hard contact lens trial are always more reliable.

Automated Keratometry

Automated keratometers are usually more accurate than manual keratometers in corneas with small optical zone (ú 3 mm) RKs because they sample a smaller central area of the cornea (nominally 2.6 mm). In addition, the automated instruments often have additional eccentric fixation targets that provide more information about the paracentral cornea. When a measurement error on an RK cornea is made, the instrument almost always gives a central corneal power that is greater than the true refractive power of the cornea. This error occurs because the samples at 2.6 mm are very close to the paracentral knee of the RK. The smaller the optical zone and the greater the number of the RK incisions, the greater the probability and magnitude of the error. Most of the automated instruments have reliability factors that are given for each measurement helping the clinician decide on the reliability in the measurement.

Automated keratometry measurements following LASIK or PRK yield accurate measurements of the front radius of the cornea because the transition areas are far outside the 2.6 mm zone that is measured. The measurements are still not accurate, however, because the assumed *net* index of refraction (4/3) is no longer appropriate for the new relationship of the front and back radius of the cornea after PRK or LASIK, just as with the topographic instruments. The *change* in central corneal power as measured by the keratometer from PRK or LASIK must be increased by 14% to determine the actual refractive change at the plane of the cornea. Hence, the automated keratometer will overestimate the power of the cornea proportional to the amount of PRK or LASIK performed.

Manual Keratometry

Manual keratometers are the least accurate in measuring central corneal power following keratorefractive procedures because the area that they measure is usually larger than automated at 3.2 mm in diameter. Therefore, measurements in this area are extremely unreliable for RK corneas with optical zones ≤ 4 mm. The one advantage with the manual keratometer is that the examiner is actually able to see the reflected mires and the amount of irregularity present. Seeing the mires does not help get a better measurement, but does allow the observer to discount the measurement as unreliable.

The manual keratometer has the same problem with PRK and LASIK as topographers and automated keratometers, and is therefore no less accurate. The manual keratometer will overestimate the change in the central refractive power of the cornea by 14% following PRK and LASIK.

■ Choosing the Desired Postoperative Refraction Target

Determining the desired postoperative refractive target is no different than other patients with cataracts in which the refractive status and the presence of a cataract in the other eye are the major determining factors. A complete discussion of avoiding refractive problems with cataract surgery is beyond the scope of this text, and is thoroughly discussed in Holladay and Rubin.[18] A short discussion of the major factors will follow.

If the patient has *binocular cataracts*, the decision is much easier because the refractive status of both eyes can be changed. The most important decision is whether the patient prefers to be myopic and read without glasses, or near emmetropic and drive without glasses. In some cases the surgeon and patient may choose the intermediate distance (-1.00 D) for the best compromise.

Targeting for monovision is certainly acceptable, provided the patient has successfully utilized monovision in the past. Trying to produce monovision in a patient who has never experienced this condition may cause intolerable anisometropia and require further surgery.

Monocular cataracts allow fewer choices for the desired postoperative refraction, because the refractive status of the other eye is fixed. The general rule is that the operative eye must be within 2 D of the nonoperative eye in order to avoid intolerable anisometropia. In most cases this means matching the other eye or targeting for up to 2 D nearer emmetropia, that is, if the unoperative eye is—5.00 D, then the target would be -3.00 D for the operative eye. If the patient is successfully wearing a contact in the unoperative eye or has already demonstrated his ability to accept monovision, then an exception can be made to the general rule. It should always be stressed, however, that should the patient be unable to continue wearing a contact, the necessary glasses for binocular correction may be intolerable and additional refractive surgery may be required.

■ Special Limitations of Intraocular Lens Power Calculation Formulas

As discussed previously, the third generation formulas (Holladay 1, Hoffer Q, and the SRK/T) and the new Holladay 2 are much more accurate than previous formulas for the more unusual eye. Older formulas such as the SRK I, SRK II, and Binkhorst I should not be used in these cases. None of these formulas will give the desired result if the central corneal power is measured incorrectly. The resulting errors are almost always in the hyperopic direction following keratorefractive surgery, because the measured corneal powers are usually greater than the true refractive power of the cornea.

To further complicate matters, the newer formulas often use keratometry as one of the predictors to estimate ELP of the intraocular lens. In patients who have had keratorefractive surgery, the corneal power is usually much flatter than normal and certainly flatter than before the keratorefractive procedure. In short, a patient with a 38.0 D cornea without keratorefractive surgery would not be expected to be similar to a patient with a 38.0 D cornea with keratorefractive surgery. Newer IOL calculation programs are now being developed to handle these situations and will improve our predictability in these cases.

■ Preoperative Evaluation

The full ophthalmologic evaluation of these patients should include a careful examination of the cornea especially in those patients who have undergone incisional keratotomy (Figs. 1–1, and 1–2). It will be important to have information about the corneal stability.[21,22]

The presence of pearls or epithelial plugs may lead to postoperative wound gaping and an unstable cornea.

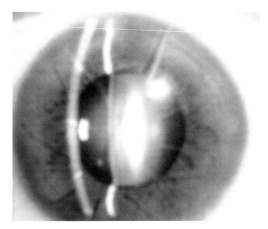

FIGURE 1–1. Cataract in patient post-radial keratotomy (RK).

■ Surgical Procedure

Wound Construction

The incision for phacoemulsification can be either clear corneal or scleral tunnel.

It may be advisable that in patients with previous incisional keratotomy to place the cataract incision between the radial incisions. Clear corneal incision may be considered in a patient with four or less radial incisions or in patients with previous PRK or LASIK. For patients with six or more radial incisions consider a scleral tunnel incision especially if the radial incisions transverse the limbus.

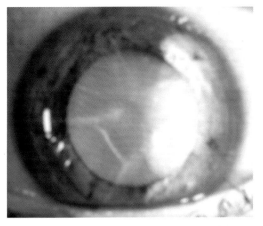

FIGURE 1–2. Cataract in patient post-RK and post-astigmatic keratotomy (AK).

Intraoperative Visualization and Corneal Protection

Intraoperative visualization is usually more difficult in patients with previous RK than in the normal cataract patient and is somewhat similar to severe arcus senilis or other conditions that cause peripheral corneal haze. The surgeon should be prepared for this additional difficulty by making sure that the patient is lined up to visualize the cataract through the optical zone. This usually means lining the microscope perpendicular to the center of the cornea, so that the surgeon is looking directly through the optical zone at the center of the cataract. When removing the peripheral cortex, the eye can be rotated so that visualization of the periphery is through the central optical zone. It is also prudent to coat the endothelium with viscoelastic to minimize any endothelial cell loss, because the keratorefractive procedure may have caused some prior loss.

Care should be taken to avoid excessive irrigation with low aspiration rate which may lead to gaping of the radial incisions.

Intraoperative Autorefractor/Retinoscopy

Large refractive surprises can be avoided by intraoperative retinoscopy or hand-held autorefractors. These refractions should not be relied upon, however, for fine tuning the intraocular lens power because there are many factors at surgery that may change in the postoperative period. Factors such as the pressure from the lid speculum, axial position of the intraocular lens, intraocular pressure, etc., may cause the intraoperative refraction to be different than the final stabilized postoperative refraction. If the intraoperative refraction is within 2 D of the target refraction, no lens exchanges should be considered unless intraoperative keratometry can also be performed.

■ Postoperative Evaluation

Refraction on the First Postoperative Day

On the first postoperative day following cataract surgery, patients who previously have had RK usually have a hyperopic shift similar to the first postoperative day following their RK. This phenomenon is primarily due to the transient corneal edema that usually exaggerates the RK effect. These patients also exhibit the same daily fluctuations during the early postoperative period after their cataract surgery as they did after the RK. Usually this daily shift is in a myopic direction during the day due to the regression of corneal edema after awakening in the morning.[19] Because the refractive changes are expected and vary significantly among patients, no lens exchange should be contemplated until after the first postoperative week or until after the refraction has stabilized, whichever is longer (Figs. 1–3 and 1–4).

Very few results of cataract surgery following PRK and LASIK are available. In the few cases that have been performed, the hyperopic shift on the first day and daily fluctuations appear to be much less, similar to the early postoperative period following these procedures. In most cases the stability of the cornea makes these cases no different than patients that have not had keratorefractive surgery.

Long-term Results

Long-term results of cataract surgery following RK are very good. The long-term hyperopic shifts and development of against-the-rule astigmatism over time following cataract surgery should be the same as in the long-term studies following RK. The problems with

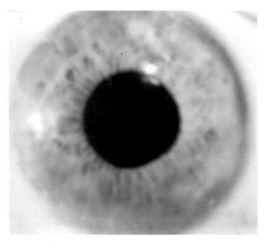

FIGURE 1–3. Postop Phaco in a patient with previous RK.

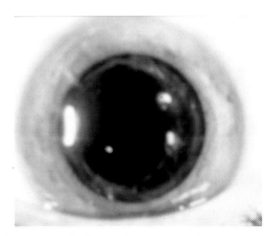

FIGURE 1–4. Postop Phaco in a patient with previous RK.

glare and starburst patterns are usually minimal because the patients have had to adjust to these unwanted optical images following the initial RK. If the patient's primary complaint before cataract surgery is glare and starbursts, it should be made clear to the patient that only the glare due to the cataract will be removed by surgery, and the symptoms that are due to the RK will remain unchanged.

Long-term results following PRK and LASIK are nonexistent. Because there are no signs of hyperopic drifts or development of against-the-rule astigmatism in the 5 year studies following PRK, one would not expect to see these changes. However, the early studies following RK did not suggest any of these long-term changes either. Only time will tell whether central haze, irregular astigmatism, etc., will be problems that develop in the future.

■ Secondary Piggy-Back IOL Implantation to Correct Unwanted Residual Refractive Errors Following Primary Cataract Surgery (IOL Calculations Using Ks and Preoperative Refraction, Axial Length Not Required)

Formula and Rationale for Using Preoperative Refraction vs. Axial Length

In a standard cataract removal with IOL implantation, the preoperative refraction is not very helpful in calculating the power of the implant because the crystalline lens will be removed so dioptric power is being removed and then replaced. In cases where no power is being removed from the eye, such as secondary implant in aphakia, piggy-back IOL in pseudophakia or a minus IOL in the anterior chamber of a phakic patient, the necessary IOL power for a desired postoperative refraction can be calculated from the corneal power and preoperative refraction, the axial length is not necessary. The formula for calculating the necessary IOL power is given below:[20]

$$IOL = \frac{1336}{\frac{1336}{\frac{1000}{1000} - \text{DPostRs}}} - \frac{1336}{\frac{1336}{\frac{1000}{1000} - \text{DPostRs}}}$$

where ELP = expected lens position in millimeters (distance from corneal vertex to principal plane of intraocular lens); IOL = intraocular lens power in diopters; K = net corneal power in diopters; PreRx = preoperative refraction in diopters; DPostRx = desired postoperative refraction in diopters; and V = vertex distance in millimeters.

Cases in Which Calculation From Preoperative Refraction

As mentioned above, the appropriate cases for using the preoperative refraction and corneal power include (1) secondary implant in aphakia; (2) secondary piggy-back IOL in pseudophakia; and (3) a minus anterior chamber IOL in a high myopic phakic patient. In each of these cases no dioptric power is being removed from the eye, so the problem is simply to find the intraocular lens at a given distance behind the cornea ELP that is equivalent to the spectacle lens at a given vertex distance in front of the cornea. If emmetropia is not desired, then an additional term, the desired postoperative refraction (DPostRx), must be included. The formulas for calculating the predicted refraction and the back-calculation of the effective lens position ELP are given in the reference and will not be repeated here.[20]

Example: Secondary Implant for Aphakia

The patient is 72 years old, aphakic in the right eye, and pseudophakic in the left eye. The right eye can no longer tolerate an aphakic contact lens. The capsule in the right eye is intact and a posterior chamber intraocular lens is desired. The patient is -0.50 D in the left eye and would like to be the same in the right eye.

Mean Keratometric K = 45.00 D
  Aphakic Refraction = +12.00 sphere @ vertex of 14 mm
  Manufacturers ACD Lens Constant = 5.25 mm
Desired Postoperative Refraction = -0.50 D

Each of the values above can be substituted in the refraction formula above except for the Manufacturers ACD and the measured K-reading. The labeled values on intraocular lens boxes are primarily for lenses implanted in the bag. Since this lens is intended for the sulcus, 0.25 mm should be subtracted from 5.25 mm to arrive at the equivalent constant for the sulcus. The ELP is therefore 5.00 mm. The K-reading must be converted from the measured keratometric K-reading (n = 1.3375) to the net K-reading (n = 4/3), for the reasons described previously under corneal topography. The conversion is performed by multiplying the measured K-reading by the following fraction:

$$\text{Fraction} = \frac{(4/3) - 1}{1.3375 - 1} = \frac{(1/3)}{0.3375} = 0.98765$$

Mean Refractive K = Mean Keratometric K * Fraction
Mean Refractive K = 45.00 * 0.98765 = 44.44 D

Using the Mean Refractive K, aphakic refraction, vertex distance, ELP for the sulcus and the desired postoperative refraction, the patient needs a 22.90 D IOL. A 23 D intraocular lens would yield a predicted refraction of -0.57 D.[20]

Example: Secondary Piggy-Back IOL for Pseudophakia

In patients with a significant residual refractive error following the primary intraocular lens implant, it is often easier surgically and more predictable optically to leave the primary implant in place and calculate the secondary piggy-back intraocular lens power to achieve the desired refraction. This method does not require knowledge of the power of the primary implant nor the axial length.

This method is particularly important in cases where the primary implant is thought to be mislabeled. The formula works for plus or minus lenses, but negative lenses are just becoming available at this time.

The patient is 55 years old and had a refractive surprise after the primary cataract surgery and was left with a +5.00 D spherical refraction in the right eye. There is no cataract in the left eye and he is plano. The surgeon and the patient both desire him to be -0.50 D, which was the target for the primary implant. The refractive surprise is felt to be from a mislabeled intraocular lens, which is centered in-the-bag and would be very difficult to remove. The secondary piggy-back intraocular lens will be placed in the sulcus. This is very important, because trying to place the second lens in-the-bag several weeks after the primary surgery is very difficult. More importantly, it may displace the primary lens posteriorly, reducing its effective power and leaving the patient with a hyperopic error. Placing the lens in the sulcus minimizes this posterior displacement.

Mean Keratometric K = 45.00 D
Pseudophakic Refraction = +5.00 sphere @ vertex of 14 mm
Manufacturers ACD Lens Constant = 5.25 mm
Desired Postoperative Refraction = -0.50 D

Using the same style lens and constant as the previous example and modifying the K-reading to net power, the formula yields a +8.64 D intraocular lens for a -0.50 D target. The nearest available lens is +9.0 D which would result in -0.76 D. In these cases extreme care should be taken to assure that the two lenses are well centered with respect to one another. Decentration of either lens can result in poor image quality and can be the limiting factor in the patient's vision.

Example: Primary Minus Anterior Chamber IOL in a High Myopic Phakic Patient
The calculation of a minus intraocular lens in the anterior chamber is no different than the aphakic calculation of an anterior chamber lens, except the power of the lens is negative. In the past, these lenses have been reserved for high myopia that could not be corrected by RK or PRK. Since most of these lenses fixate in the anterior chamber angle, concerns of iritis and glaucoma can raised. Nevertheless, several successful cases can be performed with good refractive results. Because predictable and successful LASIK procedures have been performed in myopias up to -14.00 D, these lenses may be reserved for myopia exceeding this power in the future. Interestingly, the power of the negative anterior chamber implant is very close to the spectacle refraction for normal vertex distances.

Mean Keratometric K = 45.00 D
Phakic Refraction = -20.00 sphere @ vertex of 14 mm
Manufacturers ACD Lens Constant = 3.50 mm
Desired Postoperative Refraction = -0.50 D

Using an ELP of 3.50 and modifying the K-reading to net corneal power yields a 218.49 D for a desired refraction of 20.50 D. If a 219.00 D lens is used, the patient would have a predicted postoperative refraction of 20.10 D.

■ Tips and Pearls

1. Record seven preoperative measurements (K-readings, axial length, horizontal corneal diameter, anterior chamber depth, lens thickness, preoperative refraction, and age) to accurately determine the size of the eye.
2. Use the Holladay 2 formula, especially in unusual eyes.
3. Use piggy-back intraocular lenses to achieve dioptric powers greater than 34.
4. Beware of eyes with short axial lengths (<20 mm) and small horizontal corneal diameters (<10.5 mm), these eyes are nanophthalmic and are associated with choroidal effusion and malignant glaucoma at surgery.
5. For patients who have had refractive surgery and now need cataract surgery, always perform the Calculation Method and Trial Contact Lens Method, in addi-

tion to topography and keratometric measurements to determine the corneal power.
6. Always use the lowest reliable value for the corneal power to minimize the chance for a hyperopic error.
7. Never target the desired postoperative refraction following cataract surgery to be greater than two Diopters from the other eye, unless the second eye requires cataract surgery inmediately.
8. Protect the cornea at surgery with viscoelastic and position the eye to optimize visualization through the central cornea optical zone.
9. Utilize intraoperative retinoscopy and autorefractors to eliminate large refractive surprises in unusual cases or in cases requiring lens exchange.
10. Expect fluctuations in refraction postoperatively similar to the original refractive procedure (i.e., hyperopia on the first postoperative day with a gradual decrease over the first week).
22. Use the refraction formula and secondary piggy-back intraocular lenses to correct unwanted refractive surprises following cataract surgery, rather than lens exchange.

■ ACKNOWLEDGMENTS

Special thanks to Tadeu Cvintal, M.D., for providing the photographs for this chapter.

REFERENCES

1. Holladay JT, Prager TC, Ruiz RS, Lewis JW. Improving the predictability of intraocular lens calculations. Arch Ophthalmol 1986;104:539–541.
2. Holladay JT, Prager TC, Chandler TY, Musgrove KH, Lewis JW, Ruiz RS. A three-part system for refining intraocular lens power calculations. J Cataract Refract Surg 1988;13:17–24.
3. Fedorov SN, Kolinko AI, Kolinko AI. Estimation of optical power of the intraocular lens. Vestnk Oftalmol 1967;80:27–31.
4. Fyodorov SN, Galin MA, Linksz A. Calculation of the optical power of intraocular lenses. Invest Opthalmol 1975;14:625–628.
5. Binkhorst CD. Power of the prepupillary pseudophakos. Br J Ophthalmol 1972;56:332–337.
6. Colenbrander MC. Calculation of the power of an iris clip lens for distant vision. Br J Ophthalmol 1973;57:735–740.
7. Binkhorst RD. The optical design of intraocular lens implants. Ophthalmic Surg 1975;6:17–31.
8. Van Der Heijde GL. The optical correction of unilateral aphakia. Trans Am Acad Ophthalmol Otolaryngol 1976;81:80–88.
9. Thijssen JM. The emmetropic and the iseikonic implant lens: computer calculation of the refractive power and its accuracy. Ophthalmologica 1975;171:467–586.
10. Fritz KJ. Intraocular lens power formulas. Am J Ophthalmol 1981;91:414–415.
11. Binkhorst RD. Intraocular lens power calculation manual. A guide to the author's TI 58/59 IOL Power Module. 2nd ed. New York: Binkhorst;1981.
12. Olsen T, Corydon L, Gimbel H. Intraocular lens power calculation with an improved anterior chamber depth prediction algorithm. J Cataract Refract Surg 1995;21:313–319.
13. Holladay JT, Gills JP, Leidlein J, Cherchio M. Achieving emmetropia in extremely short eyes with two piggy-back postrior chamber intraocular lenses. Ophthalmology 1996;103:1118–1123.
14. Retzlaff JA, Sanders DR, Kraff MC. Development of the SRK/T intraocular lens implant power calculation formula. J Cataract Refract Surg 1990;16:333–340.
15. Hoffer KJ. The Hoffer Q formula: A comparison of theoretic and regression formulas. J Cataract Refract Surg 1993;19:700–712.
16. Holladay JT. IOL calculations following RK. Refract Corn Surg J 1989;5:203.
17. Lowe RF, Clark BA. Posterior corneal curvature. Br J Ophthalmol 1973;57:464–470.
18. Holladay JT, Rubin ML. Avoiding refractive problems in cataract surgery. Surv Ophthalmol 1988;32:357–360.
19. Holladay JT. Management of hyperopic shift after RK. Refract Corn Surg J 1992;8:325.
20. Holladay JT. Refractive power calculation for intraocular lenses in the phakic eye. Am J Ophthalmol 1993;116:63–66.
21. Waring GO, Steinberg EB, Wilson LA. Slit lamp microcopic appearance after corneal wound healing. Am J Ophthalmol 1985;100:218–224.
22. Fyodorov SN, Sarkizova MB, Kurasovat P. Corneal biomicroscopy following repeated radial keratotomy. Am J Ophthalmol 1983;15:403–407.
23. Holladay JT. Achieving Emmetropia in Extremely Short Eyes with Piggy-Back Posterior Chamber IOLs. ASCRS Symposium on Cataract, IOL and Refractive Surgery. Seattle, WA, June 1–5, 1996.

2

Phacoemulsification in Patients with High Myopia

PAUL S. KOCH

Cataract surgery in eyes with high myopia are among the most interesting cases we face on a regular basis. The entire gamut of our surgical skills are called into play, because these eyes may present with puzzling diagnostic challenges, interesting anatomical variances, and postoperative complications which are, in all likelihood, over exaggerated. Sharp attentiveness to the unique features of these eyes can make cataract surgery essentially routine.

■ Definition

High myopia can be defined in several ways. Prior to surgical evaluation, we can define high myopia in terms of refraction. We can also define it in terms of axial length.

Refractive high myopia is variously defined as eyes with greater than 6 or 7 D of refractive error. The refractive definition is the most commonly used in the community and is very helpful for separating those patients with significant ocular differences from those with more routine myopia. This definition is easily established and represents the initial basis for all of our discussions.

A more precise way of defining the long eye is in terms of its axial length. This allows us to isolate those eyes that are truly long from those that are normal size, but have steep corneas. Like its refractive cousin, this definition is fluid with various reports extending the threshold from 25.0 to 27.0 mm.[1-6]

■ Demographics

There are many relationships between myopia and cataract. One common one is the development of induced myopia in association with progression of a nuclear sclerotic cataract. However, on an anatomic basis, there are other relationships that help define the uniqueness of the cataract in high myopia. For example, there is a subset of individuals who demonstrate a relationship among high myopia, cataract, and youth. Kaufman and Sugar documented this relationship in a study in which they evaluated young patients with myopia who presented with a visually disabling cataract. In a group of 12 consecutive patients, the mean age was 44 years, (range 34 to 54 years).[7] DeNatale et al measured the relationship between high myopia and lens opacity using the Lens Opacity Meter 701. They compared 91 high myopia eyes with a control group of 106 emmetropic eyes. The myopia group always had higher lens opacity values and this result was statistically significant after the age of 20 years.[8]

■ Preoperative Evaluation

Diagnosis

Unlike cataracts in otherwise normal eyes, the diagnosis of cataracts in an eye with high myopia can be a challenge. They tend to be visually disabling when still quite small and can be dismissed as a cause for visual problems. O'Donnell and Maumenee discussed "unexplained" visual loss in axial myopia when caused by a mild nuclear sclerotic cataract. In patients with axial high myopia, these mild cataracts can be an unappreciated cause of visual acuity loss and are often overlooked during the diagnostic examination. These patients can have media which are far better than the visual acuity would suggest. The investigators suggest considering cataracts as the principal diagnosis when the patient's evaluation demonstrates monocular diplopia, near acuity more compatible with the media, and retinoscopic evidence of nuclear sclerosis.[9]

Kaufman and Sugar confirmed this with observations that patients with high myopia can present with a progressive decrease in vision, or with disabling monocular polyopia. In their study, presumed diagnoses ranged from keratoconus to myopic degeneration. Presence of a cataract was frequently overlooked. Cataract extraction was therapeutic and its prompt diagnosis can eliminate unnecessary testing and repeated office visits.[7]

Case Report: A 52-year-old woman presented to our clinic with gradual loss of visual acuity in both eyes. Her life-long refraction of approximately −7.00 had not changed and her best corrected visual acuity of 20/50 at distance was a significant drop from her previous 20/20. Her near acuity was similar to her distance. The eye examination appeared completely normal. The lenses were clear. Over the next 10 months, her vision slowly declined to 20/100. She had a thorough work-up, including multiple examinations, perimetry, fluorescein angiography, and neuro-imaging. At all times the eye appeared normal and the lens clear. Eventually, she complained of several other symptoms, including difficulty driving at night and glare, which sounded like classic cataract symptoms. We weighed the possibility that she had an "invisible cataract," which is sometimes found in patients with high myopia. We discussed this potential scenario with her and together decided to proceed with cataract surgery. By the following day, her vision had improved to 20/20 and symptoms in that eye were resolved. Successful surgery was performed in the other eye a few weeks later.

Retina Evaluation

The peripheral retina needs to be evaluated prior to surgery so that potential risk factors for retinal detachment can be identified and treated if necessary. If the peripheral retina is easily examined, this can be done by the surgeon, but in cases where the examination is challenging, the assistance of a retinal specialist may be appreciated.

IOL Calculation

Biometry and calculation of a lens (IOL) implant is sometimes difficult. Eyes with normally rounded posterior segments are not usually a problem, but eyes with staphylomas are. The point of foveal fixation can be at the top edge of the staphyloma, on its slope, or at its base. Repeated examinations with the patient focused on the tip of the biometry probe is one way to establish the axial length of the refractive system, as opposed to the maximum size of the eye. B-scan ultrasonography is also useful in some cases in which the biometry is difficult to map out the shape of the posterior segment and to assist the biometer to determine the approximate placement of the visual center.

All old intraocular lens (IOL) calculation programs are hopelessly inaccurate when dealing with long eyes. The theoretical formulas which compensate for the length of the eye, including the relative increased length of the anterior segment are better. The theoretical formulas most commonly used are the SRK-T (not the SRK or the SRK II), the Holladay, and the Hoffer-Q.

Surgical Procedure

Anesthesia

All traditional methods of anesthesia can be used successfully in long eyes, but there is a danger of globe perforation when a retrobulbar injection is given. Ramsay and Knobloch reported that in a series of 4000 consecutive patients who had retrobulbar anesthesia, three of them had globe perforation. In all three cases, significant myopia was present. In order to avoid this potential complication, anesthetic methods that do not require retrobulbar injection are often used.

Gills (presentation Annual Meeting, American Academy of Ophthalmology, Atlanta, GA, 1995) suggested the use of intraocular lidocaine as an adjunct to topical anesthesia. The topical agent is used prior to surgery to anesthetize the cornea. A stab incision is made in the peripheral cornea and 0.5 cc of 1% unpreserved lidocaine is irrigated into the anterior chamber. The effect is almost instantaneous and lasts for at least 30 minutes. Intraocular anesthesia is a very safe and effective way to anesthetize any eye prior to cataract surgery, but especially safe in patients with high myopia.

If a corneal incision is used this technique does not have to be modified at all. If, however, a conjunctival flap is raised in preparation for a scleral tunnel incision, this anesthesia is not always adequate in preventing discomfort during cauterization of bleeding scleral vessels. If cautery is necessary, it is helpful to place a few drops of a topical agent on the sclera prior to cauterization.[10]

Incision

Making an incision and developing access to the anterior chamber is usually very easy in eyes with myopia, because of their size. The relative exophthalmos of a highly myopic eye causes the anterior segment to sit up like a golf ball on a tee. There is much greater exposure for surgery than with normal-sized eyes. The extra exposure facilitates surgery from either the top or from the side. My preference is to perform each cataract operation using a temporal corneal incision, which is 2.65 mm wide. Many eyes with high myopia, however, require longer incisions. This is because they need a very low plus-powered lens, or sometimes a minus-powered lens. These lenses are all available only as rigid polymethylmethacrylate lenses and will not fit through the small phaco incision. In these cases, the incision has to be opened several millimeters for lens insertion and then sutured afterwards.

Once the nucleus is pushed back, either from viscoelastic or from infusion, the distance from the incision to the cataract increases. The phaco tip and all other instruments have to be angled more vertically than usual. In order to accommodate this, the incision entry into the eye needs to be close to the periphery of the cornea and the tunnel should not be too long. If an extremely long tunnel with a large corneal valve is created, it is very difficult to tilt the instruments toward the cataract without distorting the cornea significantly. A more traditional and conservative incision makes instrument manipulation much simpler. It is not necessary that the incision entry be very peripheral, only one that is not extreme in the other direction.

Hydrodissection

Because these patients are typically younger than the average cataract patient, there are usually very strong adhesions in the interface connecting nucleus, epinucleus, cortex, and capsule. In order to minimize trauma to the capsular bag, it is critical that these adhesions be broken prior to nucleus manipulation. Thorough and vigorous hydrodissection should be used to free up the cataract entirely, thereby facilitating its separation and removal. Efforts should be made to perform complete cortical cleaving hydrodissection, separating all of the cortex from the capsule in order to minimize any tension on the capsule whatsoever during nucleus rotation and removal.

Nucleus Removal

When removing the nucleus, the preferred technique is phacoemulsification followed by nucleus expression extracapsular surgery, leaving intracapsular surgery as the last resort. Phacoemulsification maintains a relatively stable pressure in the anterior chamber during the operation and this tamponades the posterior capsule. Wild fluctuations in anterior chamber pressure can cause a posterior capsule to bounce and this can permit disturbances in the vitreous. Long eyes already have a tenuous vitreous base and everything that can be done to maintain its structural integrity is helpful in the long run.

A practical consideration in phacoemulsification is the fact that these eyes are quite large and the anterior chambers are deep. When performing phacoemulsification, it is only necessary to move the tip a little deeper into the eye, and with the instrument angled slightly more vertically, the nucleus can be emulsified using standard techniques. The extra millimeter or two of distance is of little consequence. On the other hand, removing the nucleus using an expression technique is a bit challenging. The nucleus has to be lifted out of the capsular bag and then an additional distance to get it to the incision. This requires either additional manipulation within the anterior chamber, or additional pressure on the globe in order to transmit positive vitreous pressure against the back of the posterior capsule. This leads to a rather extreme difference in ocular pressures, with the high vitreous pressure pushing the nucleus into the very low pressure of the anterior chamber and extraocular environment. This imbalance is to be avoided whenever possible, for reasons mentioned above. Obviously, the extreme case of removing the posterior capsule entirely using an intracapsular technique is to be avoided whenever possible.

Because patients with high myopia and cataracts tend to be young, the cataract appears to be soft. The nuclear sclerotic component is reasonably transparent. The brown discoloration seen in older patients is typically not present. As a result, the red reflex is usually quite bright. When phacoemulsification is begun, a common error is to be deceived by this appearance and assume the cataract is soft. Actually, these cataracts are frequently more dense than the appearance would suggest. It is important to use sufficient phaco power when sculpting because the red reflex alone would suggest that only a little energy is needed (Fig. 2–1). If insufficient power is used, the nucleus will not be cut, but will rock back-and-forth in the capsular bag. This will traumatize not only the bag, but the zonules, and can lead to capsular tear or zonular dehiscence. This is to be avoided at all costs. Cataracts in eyes with high myopia require surprisingly high energy levels, at least when performing initial sculpting. Later in the operation, when performing nucleus segment removal, adequate phaco powers are generally used, because by this time the surgeon has established the nucleus density and critical parameters necessary for easy emulsification (Fig. 2–2).

Pupillary Dilation

Pupillary dilation in high myopia is a little different than in other eyes. These eyes tend to dilate only moderately, but this is a temporary

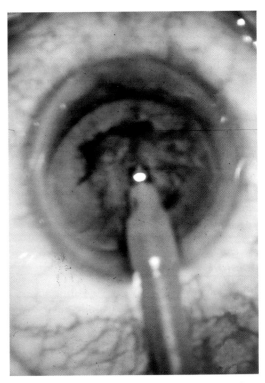

FIGURE 2–1. Phacoemulsification in a high myope. (Photo provided by Dr. Luis W. Lu)

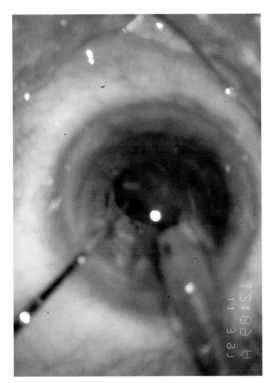

FIGURE 2–2. Removal with adequate phaco parameters. (Photo provided by Dr. Luis W. Lu)

rior capsule during the operation is a very high priority, but that is not enough. The rigid barrier of an intraocular lens is necessary to resist all efforts of the vitreous to come forward. For many years, we in the U.S. have been handicapped by the lack of availability of low-powered lenses. When faced with a patient with high myopia, our choices were to use the lowest available lens, which frequently left the patient extremely nearsighted following surgery, or to try to achieve a better refractive result and put in no lens whatsoever. Happily, this dilemma has been resolved with the new availability of lenses down to −18.0 D, which ought to satisfy the needs of any eye. These lenses are one-piece PMMA lenses, so they require a 6 mm incision (Figs. 2–3 to 2–6).

At the present time, we don't have a lot of choice in the matter because of the limited design availability, but as a rule long eyes are also wide ones. Intraocular lenses should be available with large diameter optics, to fill the large capsular bag and hide behind the large pupil. Haptic length should be longer than average for best fit. Great care should be de-

phenomenon. Once the phaco tip is introduced into the eye and irrigation activated, the anterior chamber pressure increases. This pushes the nucleus back, taking pressure off the iris diaphragm. As the iris falls back, the pupil dilates, frequently by an extra millimeter or two. This improves visualization for much of the procedure. The same phenomenon occurs when the anterior chamber is filled with a viscoelastic pushing the nucleus and iris back. The increase in pupil dilation improves visualization for capsulorhexis and for emulsification. Unfortunately, as the intraocular pressure varies during surgery, so does the pupillary diameter. As the lens/iris diaphragm moves up and down in response to pressure variation, the pupil size changes as well. Unless the irrigation and aspiration are perfectly balanced, the pupil will seem to "breathe" as the case progresses.

Preserving a Barrier

It is extremely important to maintain a barrier within the eye to provide stability to the entire posterior segment. Preservation of the poste-

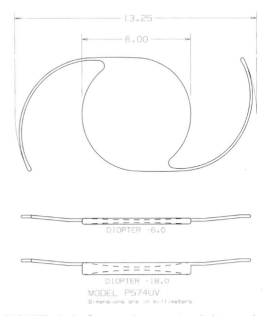

FIGURE 2–3. Storz minus-powered intraocular lens, Model P574UV. At −6.0 D the lens is very thin with the bi-concave meniscus removed from its center. As the power becomes progressively stronger (i.e., more minus), the optic edge has to be thicker to accommodate the more pronounced concavity.

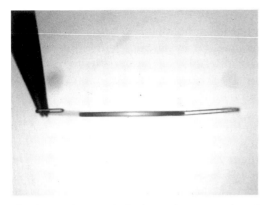

FIGURE 2–4. −6.00 D lens demonstrating its thinness in profile.

voted to preserving the capsular bag, because some eyes are so large that a typical posterior chamber lens will not anchor in the sulcus. Anterior chamber lenses, if needed, will often spin rather than fixate, as we are accustomed to seeing.

■ Postoperative Considerations

Postoperative Refraction

The most significant refractive problem following any elective operation is induced hyperopia. There is never a degree of hyperopia which is beneficial to a patient. Unless a patient is brought there to balance a fellow eye, postoperative refraction should be planned to be either emmetropic or myopic. In the case

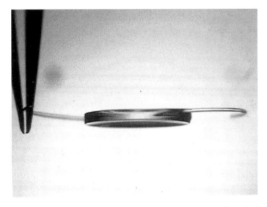

FIGURE 2–5. −18.00 D lens demonstrating it is relatively thicker in order to accomodate the more pronounced concavity.

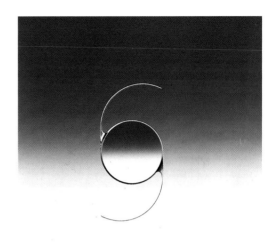

FIGURE 2–6. −18.00 D intraocular lens (Storz P574).

of high myopia, the decision-making process is a bit complicated.

If a patient has a cataract in only one eye and typically wears contact lens, it is possible to seek a postoperative result close to emmetropia because the eyes will balance well. If the patient is wearing spectacles, discussion must be undertaken to determine whether the patient would be best served by leaving the one cataract eye myopic, otherwise anisometropia will develop. The alternative in these patients is to seek a refraction close to emmetropia, with the understanding that the other eye will also have surgery in order to balance the pair.

Kora et al pooled 84 patients with high myopia who had had cataract surgery about their preferences for postoperative vision. Once certain tasks were defined, each patient was fitted with contact lenses to render them either emmetropic, −3.00 D myopic, or −5.00 D myopic. Among those patients with vision of at least 20/40, 86% preferred either emmetropia (38%) or −3.00 D of myopia (48%). Among those patients with best-corrected vision worse than 20/200, 80% preferred the −5.00 D of myopia because of the reading magnification it provided. They found that patients with good visual potential appreciated overall distance vision, but those with low potential preferred near magnification. Certainly it is important to take patient preference into consideration when selecting the target postoperative refraction.[11]

Complications

The well-known horror stories about the complications in cataract surgery in eyes with high myopia were to a large degree based on intracapsular cataract surgery (ICCE). Extracapsular cataract extraction (ECCE) of all sorts, is much safer. Jaffe et al reported a reduction in the incidence of postoperative retinal detachment in long eyes from 5.74% with ICCE, to 0.66% with ECCE.[12] Other reports confirm the rate of retinal detachment following ECCE to be less than 2%.[2–5,13–15]

Another feared complication is a acute suprachoroidal hemorrhage. Hoffman et al detailed a correlation between limited choroidal hemorrhage occurring following ICCE and pre-operative myopia. In a study of 521 eyes, 16 (13.07%) had evidence of a limited choroidal hemorrhage. It occurred in 14.9% of highly myopic eyes, 4.5% of moderately myopic eyes, and 0.77% of eyes without clinically significant myopia.[16]

Interestingly, there is a frequently reported complication that has clinical significance for a number of patients in the postoperative period. Eyes with high myopia, possibly because of the younger age group associated with cataract surgery, have a significant rate of posterior capsule opacification. In a paper on refractive lens surgery Lyle and Jin commented that posterior capsule opacification was the major complication and it developed faster than reported in other studies.[15] In another paper, they report a 50% incidence within 27 months.[3] In a paper on minus-powered IOLs, Kohnen and Brauweiler report rapid posterior capsule opacification in 14 of 32 eyes (44%).[17]

Rapid opacification of the posterior capsule has importance because of the inevitability of a capsulotomy in these eyes. This will disturb the natural physical barrier in the eye and can predispose to retinal detachment and other complications.[3] This underscores the importance of implanting intraocular lens to preserve as much barrier as possible.

■ Conclusion

One of the biggest challenges facing us when dealing with a patient with a cataract and high myopia is making the correct diagnosis in the first place. Often these cataracts appear less dense than the symptoms would suggest. Accurate diagnosis can spare the patient unnecessary time wasted between presentation and treatment, and it can avoid many unnecessary tests.

Surgery is generally proceeded by a noninjection method of anesthesia, such as irrigating the anterior chamber with 0.5 cc of 1% unpreserved lidocaine. The anterior chamber pressure should be maintained with phacoemulsification, both to avoid trauma to the vitreous and to maintain a fixed-pupil diameter. The distance the cataract sits from the cornea is a challenge, partially compensated by the relative exophthalmos and excellent exposure.

Patients with eyes with excellent vision potential tend to prefer a postoperative refraction between emmetropia and −3.00 D of myopia. If the potential is worse than 20/200, many patients prefer −5.00 D of myopia for the reading magnification effect.

Significant complications, such as retinal detachment and choroidal hemorrhage, are limited when extracapsular techniques are used. Posterior capsule opacification occurs quickly in many patients—possibly because of their young ages. The inevitability of a capsulotomy in many eyes can be anticipated and potential complications controlled by implanting an intraocular lens to maintain ocular integrity and to establish a physical barrier to prevent vitreous prolapse after the capsulotomy.

If the various unique features of cataract surgery in eyes with high myopia are kept in mind, cataract surgery can proceed as smoothly as in a more routine case. Postoperative care and complications can also be very close to the norm for emmetropic eyes.

■ Tips and Pearls

1. Consider the diagnosis of cataract when evaluating vision loss in a patient with

high myopia, even if the lens is only mildly opacified.
2. Evaluate the peripheral retina, either by yourself or with the assistance of a retinal consultant.
3. Calculate the lens power using one of the theoretical formulas.
4. Use a noninjection method of anesthesia.
5. Make the incision a little more peripheral than usual.
6. Thorough and vigorous hydrodissection.
7. Use phacoemulsification to stabilize the anterior chamber.
8. Remember to use more phaco power during sculpting than you would expect based on the brightness of the red reflex. These cataracts are more dense than they appear.
9. Maintain a physical barrier by preserving the posterior capsule and by implanting an IOL in the bag.
10. Plan the postoperative refraction based on the patient's needs and visual potential.

REFERENCES

1. Rozsival P, Kana V. Implantation of intraocular lenses in myopia. Cesk Slov Oftalmol 1996;52(2):104–108.
2. Nissen KR, Fuchs HJ, Goldschmidt E, et al. Risk of cataract surgery in patients with myopia. Ugeskr Laeger 1994;10;156(41):6014–6018.
3. Lyle WA, Jin GJ. Phacoemulsification with intraocular lens implantation in high myopia. J Cataract Refract Surg 1996;22(2):238–242.
4. Lamrani M, Korobelnik JF, Renard G, Pouliquen Y. Cataract surgery in patients with myopia. J Fr Ophtalmol 1993;16(8–9):458–463.
5. Percival SP. Redefinition of high myopia: the relationship of axial length measurement to myopic pathology and its relevance to cataract surgery. Dev Ophthalmol 1987;14:42–46.
6. Ochi T, Gon A, Kora Y, Kawai K, Fukado Y. Intraocular lens implantation and high myopia. J Cataract Refract Surg 1988;14(4):403–408.
7. Kaufman BJ, Sugar J. Discrete nuclear sclerosis in young patients with myopia. Arch Ophthalmol 1996;114(10):1178–1180.
8. De Natale R, Romeo G, Fama F, Scullica L. Human lens transparence in high-myopic subjects. Ophthalmologica 1992;205(1):7–9.
9. O'Donnell FE Jr, Maumenee AE. "Unexplained" visual loss in axial myopia: cases caused by mild nuclear sclerotic cataract. Ophthalmic Surg 1980;11(2):99–101.
10. Koch PS. Intraocular Anesthesia. Simplifying Phacoemulsification 5th Ed. Thorofare, NJ: Slack; 1997; 13–20.
11. Kora Y, Yaguchi S, Inatomi M, Ozawa T. Preferred postoperative refraction after cataract surgery for high myopia. J Cataract Refract Surg 1995;21(1):35–38.
12. Jaffe NS, Clayman HM, Jaffe MS. Retinal detachment in myopic eyes after intracapsular and extracapsular cataract extraction. Am J Ophthalmol 1984;97(1):48–52.
13. Yang WH. Extracapsular cataract extraction for highly myopic patients. Chung Hua Yen Ko Tsa Chih 1990;26(6):337–339.
14. Dong X, Xie L, Zhang Y. A clinical observation on intraocular lens implantation in high myopic eyes with cataract. Chung Hua Yen Ko Tsa Chih 1995;31(4):268–270.
15. Lyle WA, Jin GJ. Clear lens extraction for the correction of high refractive error. J Cataract Refract Surg 1994;20(3):273–276.
16. Hoffman P, Pollack A, Oliver M. Limited choroidal hemorrhage associated with intracapsular cataract extraction. Arch Ophthalmol 1984;102(12):1761–1765.
17. Kohnen S, Brauweiler P. First results of cataract surgery and implantation of negative power intraocular lenses in highly myopic eyes. J Cataract Refract Surg 1996;22(4):416–420.

3

Phacoemulsification in High Hyperopic Cataract Patients

JAMES P. GILLS AND MYRA CHERCHIO

The highly hyperopic patient presents the cataract surgeon with two potential problems. The first is the possibility of surgical complications that may arise from the structural nature of the hyperopic eye. The second is implanting adequate power while maintaining good optical quality and an accurate refraction.

Patients with short axial lengths often have very small anterior segments. About 20% of eyes with axial length less than 21 mm have disproportionately small anterior segment sizes.[1] In cases with shallow anterior chambers, we are less able to utilize clear corneal incisions (CCIs) because 2.5 mm takes up more area in a small cornea. Phacoemulsification is more challenging in a short eye. One of the challenges that may arise during phacoemulsification is pupillary block. Increased intraocular pressure (IOP) from choroidal effusion or fluid misdirection is more common in hyperopic eyes and can cause a progressive shallowing of the anterior chamber as the eye hardens. Short eyes are at greater risk for expulsive hemorrhage. Another complication associated with a short eye is iris prolapse when the phaco tip is inserted. Patients with short eyes are at increased risk of angle closure glaucoma. There are good surgical strategies which can be used to surmount these problems (see the *Surgical Management* section).

Predicting and fitting the correct intraocular lens (IOL) power in highly hyperopic patients is even more challenging due to IOL technology constraints and the limitations of current power formulas. Empirically derived power formulas were developed on normal eyes and by their nature are much less accurate for shorter and longer eyes. Current theoretical formulas have been improved enormously, providing fairly accurate power predictions for average and for moderately short and long eyes.[2-6] Nevertheless, these formulas still use empirically derived constants and estimates of optical relationships that remain more accurate for average or near-average length eyes, making power determination for high hyperopes much less predictable. Furthermore, even when the surgeon is fairly confident of the calculated power, a lens of that power is often not commercially available. Highly hyperopic patients often require substantially higher power than the 34 D which is generally the upper limit of IOL power inventories. Microphthalmic eyes may require as much as 60 D of power in the IOL plane to provide a reasonable refraction. Even if the patient and surgeon are willing to tolerate delays, bureaucracy, and added expense, custom making higher powered lenses poses tedious FDA-related problems concerning optical issues with high powered lenses. At high dioptric powers (over about 40 D), significant spherical aberrations occur. Such high powers require very steep radii, causing the lens to be shaped more like a sphere. The modulation transfer function is decreased. Thus resolution is compromised, with a severely distorted image quality.[7,8]

Because of these problems in predicting and providing adequate power for the high hyperope, severe undercorrection has often been the expected outcome. Better surgical technique, improved phacoemulsification technology and better IOL designs have given us confidence in avoiding surgical complications in the hyperopic eye. The next step is to address the power issues. A practical solution to the problem of providing accurate power for the patient with a short eye is to implant *two* IOLs piggy-back style which together provide adequate power without any compromise in optical quality. Johnny Gayton first reported implantation of two IOLs in a case of extreme microphthalmos in 1993.[9] I have applied this strategy since 1993 to less extreme cases of hyperopia in which a single high power IOL would not have provided sufficient power and even to cases in which the required power was at or near the upper limit of power inventories.[10] I implant two IOLs in these cases because when the optical centers of the lenses are aligned, they provide better optical quality than a single high powered IOL. Good refractive and visual outcomes have been documented for hyperopes receiving double (and triple) implants.[10,11]

■ General Guidelines: Preoperative Measurements, Power Calculation and Patient Strategies

Axial Length Measurement

Accurate measurement of axial length and corneal curvature have always been the starting point for obtaining predictable refractive outcome. Used in conjunction with an appropriate power calculation formula and optimized constants (specific to both the IOL and the surgeon), accurate measurements result in good outcomes in the majority of cases.[2-4] Accurate measurement of axial length in hyperopic eyes is especially important since any error is greatly magnified in proportion to the length of the eye. Yet it is in short eyes that accurate measurements are most difficult to obtain. Ultrasound axiometers are calibrated with average velocities for normal length eyes. These are incorrect for short eyes, causing significant measurement errors.[7] Performing applanation biometry is frequently difficult in short-eye cases with a shallow anterior chamber because it can be difficult to distinguish the initial "bang" echo from the iris and establish perpendicularity. Decreasing the ultrasound gain may be necessary when this occurs so each echo can be visualized but this can make the scan more difficult to perform. The most significant problem with applanation biometry is that the cornea is easily indented even in the hand of the most skilled ultrasound technician. Even the slightest indentation can cause significant measurement errors which are magnified when the eye is short.[2,7,12] For this reason I prefer immersion biometry which I believe gives superior results in these cases.[13] First, it is impossible to applanate the cornea. Thus, by its very nature, immersion is more reliable. Second, it allows visualization of the corneal echoes. In order to obtain the most accurate measurement, the skilled ultrasound technician will watch for consistency of echo height, axial length, lens thickness, and anterior chamber depth readings.

Power Calculation

Optimizing axial length measurements does not guarantee the desired outcome. In a study performed with Dr. Jack Holladay,[7] several hyperopic patients were examined and more detailed anatomical measurements were taken. In most cases the short eye cases had normal anterior segment dimensions (corneal diameter, keratometry, and anterior segment length.) The abnormality was a foreshortened

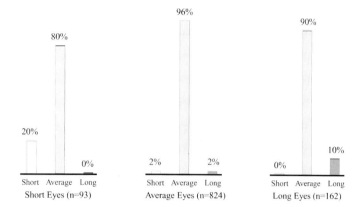

FIGURE 3–1. Distribution of anterior segment size by axial length. Note that the majority of short axial length eyes have normal anterior segment sizes. Adapted from Holladay.[1]

axial length due to a shortened posterior segment. Based on these observations we can conclude that current third generation power formulas *systematically* generate hyperopic errors in power calculation among most short eye cases because they shorten the expected anterior chamber depth to the lens as a function of the axial length.[7] Thus they all predict the position of the lens to be too far anterior, resulting in a hyperopic error. We've collaborated with Dr. Holladay in his recent multi-site study of power calculation in long and short eyes. This further work[1] has suggested that there are different types of eyes with respect to axial length and anterior segment size. About 80% of short eyes have normal anterior segment length while only 20% have short anterior segment sizes (Fig. 3–1). Figure 3–2 (A and B) shows the A-scans for two eyes with near-equivalent axial length, but with very different corneal diameters and anterior chamber depth (ACD). Thus they have very different anterior segment eyes. Examination of the relationship between predicted power (using current methods) and axial length for large, normal, and small anterior segment sizes (Fig. 3–3) shows that predicted emmetropia power is lower for short eyes.[1] Holladay estimates that short axial length cases with normal anterior segment length and shortened posterior segment length may comprise about 80% of short eyes and 0.6% of all cataract cases (see Fig. 3–1, Table 3–1).[1] This would be approximately 7200 cases per year (of about 1.2 million IOL cases)

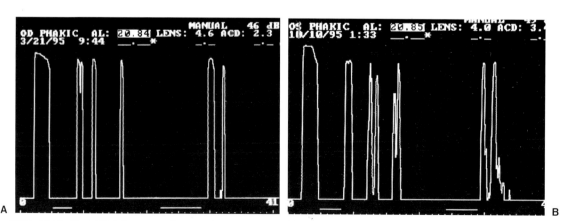

FIGURE 3–2. (Gills) A-scan printouts for two eyes with near-equivalent axial lengths but different anterior segment sizes. **(A)** The axial length is 20.84 mm while corneal diameter is 10.0 and ACD is 2.3. **(B)** The axial length is 20.85 mm but the corneal diameter is 11.0 and the ACD is 3.4. Power for the eye with the larger anterior segment would actually be less accurately predicted using current formulas.

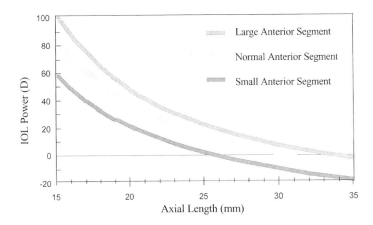

FIGURE 3–3. Schematic illustration of predicted emmetropia power (using current theoretic formulas) versus axial length for small, normal and large anterior segment sizes. Adapted from Holladay.[1]

who would receive underestimated IOL power. A new Holladay power formula has been developed on almost 1000 eyes in this study (including 93 eyes with short axial length).[1] It appears that white-to-white corneal diameter and lens thickness can be used along with anterior chamber depth to determine the size of the anterior segment and that all are important considerations for power calculation. These measurements help predict the exact location of the IOL in the short eye and increase prediction accuracy. Holladay has reported that prediction accuracy in short eyes is significantly improved in the new Holladay 2 formula, which utilizes these extra measurements.[1] He reported a decrease in mean absolute error among short eye cases from about 4.5 D when current formulas are used to a little less than 1 D when the new Holladay 2 formula is used. About 4% of eyes with *average* total axial lengths have anterior segment sizes which are large or small relative to the posterior segment (Fig. 3–1) and may also benefit from the use of a power formula based on more measurements.

Furthermore, when the piggyback technique is used in high hyperopes, power calculations must be adjusted again. By measuring the distance from the iris to the intraocular lens vertex, Holladay and Gills[12] determined that the anterior-most lens is in the usual position while the posterior-most lens is pushed back. This causes additional hyperopic error. Apparently the anterior lens pushes the posterior lens further back due to the elastic nature of the capsular bag. Because of this, additional power must be factored into the equation. The new Holladay 2 formula provides such adjustments.[1]

Patient Selection and Strategies

When axial length is short, further measurements help us to make better predictions of the necessary IOL power. Classifying patients accordingly allows us to optimize refractive and visual outcome. We can better manage patient expectations regarding refractive outcome and, in fact, provide high hyperopes with better vision than they've ever had. IOL power becomes more predictable and thus less of a limiting factor in visual outcome. Benefits derived from surgical strategies to correct preexisting astigmatism and providing fast visual recovery through the use of intraoperative anesthesia are no longer overshadowed by unpredictable power calculation. In short, the

TABLE 3–1. Distribution of Axial Length vs. Anterior Segment Size in General Population

	Axial Length		
Anterior Segment Size	Short	Normal	Long
Large	0.0%	2.0%	0.1%
Normal	0.6%	94.1%	1.1%
Small	0.1%	2.0%	0.0%

Adapted from Holladay[1]

high hyperope can expect excellent refractive and visual outcome along with average axial length patients.

■ Patient and Surgeon Preparation

Anesthesia

All patients undergoing cataract surgery receive a thorough explanation of the type of anesthesia to be used, what to expect during surgery, and the risks involved with surgery. This is especially important with high hyperopes since compliance during surgery is critical. I prefer to use topical anesthesia supplemented by preservative-free intraocular lidocaine for these patients, just as I do for cases with average axial lengths. I've found that this technique is very safe and provides the vast majority of patients with an excellent degree of comfort and speedy physical and visual recovery.[14] With proper preoperative screening and counseling, high hyperopes may also enjoy these benefits safely. Patients are highly motivated with the expectation of "pain-free" surgery and fast visual recovery. A summary of general preoperative and intraoperative medication regimens is given in Table 3–2. I find that preparing the patient psychologically for surgery can reduce the possibility of complications resulting from lid squeezing,

TABLE 3–2. Preop, Surgical, and Recovery Room Regimens

Pre-op: (exam area and again in pre-op holding area, 15 minutes prior to transfer to O.R.)
Proparacaine   0.5% 1 gtt × 2
Marcaine (without Epi.) 0.75% 1 gtt × 4 (3 min apart)
Ocuflox/Indomethacin solution 1.0% 1 gtt × 1
Preparation: Using a 5 ml bottle of Ocuflox, withdraw 1 ml to reconstitute a 1 mg vial Indomethacin. Withdraw the 1 ml Ocuflox/1 mg Indomathacin solution and add to the remaining 4 ml Ocuflox.
O.R.:
Proparacaine   0.5% 1 gtt × 2
Marcaine   0.75% 1 gtt × 4 (3 min apart with final gtt instilled just prior to start)
Ocuflox   1 gtt at case end
Intraocular Xylocaine 1%: (preservative free, without epinephrine)
0.5 ml is used prophylactically during hydrodissection to minimize patient discomfort.
Irrigation Solution:
Supplies
Heparin 1000 units/ml
Epinephrine 1:1000
Vancomycin 50 mg/ml
500 ml bottle BSS
Preparation:
To 500 ml bottle BSS add:
0.8 ml Heparin   (800 units)
0.5 ml Epinephrine   (1:1000)
0.1 ml Vancomycin   (5 mg)
A 0.22 μmicropore filter is used to filter all irrigation solutions.
(#A5900) Surgin 1-(800) 753–7400 Tustin, CA
Pre & Post-op Anterior Chamber Injection of Indomethacin and Solucortef
Draw up 15 ml BSS injecting 13 ml into an empty sterile bottle.
Use the remaining 2 ml to reconstitute two 1 mg vials of Indomethacin.
Add both of the 1 ml vials of Indomethacin solution to the 13 ml bottle of BSS.
Add 8 gtts of Solucortef 125 mg/ml (8 minims using TB syringe) to the 15 ml bottle of Indomethacin solution.
Add 0.04 ml Amikacin 100 mg/2 ml to the vial (2 mg)
Dosage per patient: 0.25ml into the A/C following initial incision then 0.25 ml again at the end of the case.
Recovery Room:
Proparacaine   0.5% 1 gtt upon arrival
Marcaine   0.75% 1 gtt × 3
Ocuflox   1 gtt × 1
Pilocarpine   1% 1 gtt × 1

Ibuprofen (200 mg) is given, 1 tab p.o preoperatively and 1 tab postoperatively unless contraindicated.

poor cooperation, etc. However, managing complications is certainly more difficult under topical anesthesia and high hyperopes are at greater risk for certain complications such as elevated IOP from fluid misdirection, iris prolapse, etc., as mentioned earlier. Other surgeons may prefer regional anesthesia for these cases.

Managing Expectations

It is important to manage patients' expectations. Frequently hyperopia is accompanied by amblyopia and the patient must be aware of the possibility of a limited improvement in vision. It is wise to test potential acuity in these cases. The amblyopic patient should be aware of the potential visual limitations. However, we've observed that often amblyopic patients report following surgery that their vision is better than it ever has been. If the patient is undergoing surgery for the first time, I also explain the probability of a severe anisometropia problem. Rather than "balancing" the first eye for a less optimal result I suggest to the patient that both eyes be operated within several days to correct the anisometropia and avoid the need for full-time glasses. If the patient is pseudophakic and underpowered in the contralateral eye, I suggest that a second IOL be implanted in the underpowered eye to provide the needed additional power. This is a major indication for the use of piggyback IOLs. The residual hyperopic error can be corrected by this method, under topical anesthesia. There is no need to do a removal/exchange which would be traumatic and is associated with posterior or anterior capsule rupture. With a damaged capsule there is decreased capsular support. Other risks increased during a removal are retinal tears, cystoid macular edema, and cyclodialysis. All this can be avoided while still correcting the residual hyperopia if the secondary piggy-back strategy is employed.

With current power formulas, there is still the possibility of underpowering the eye with a very short axial length even when double implants are used. The patient must be made aware of the possibility that an exchange of the anterior-most IOL may be necessary. One significant benefit of topical anesthesia is that the patient may be refracted immediately or on the next day to determine if an exchange is necessary. The early exchange of the IOL (sometimes on the same day) is uneventful without the risks of removal discussed earlier. The patient is left with an optimal refraction. Power "surprises" even among high hyperopes, are becoming less common as we learn more about power calculation in these cases.

IOL Selection and Surgical Procedure

All patients requiring 34 or more diopters of IOL power are given double implants. At this time we are using the Holladay 2 formula. We had been using the original Holladay formula. Never use an empirical formula (regression-based) for short eye cases. They are much less accurate than theoretical formulas.[2,3,5,6] Even if you use a current third generation theoretical formula you will have to add additional power. We added 2–3 D to the formula-predicted value before we switched to the new Holladay 2 formula. The total required power can be divided equally between the 2 IOLs. Some surgeons prefer placing 2/3 of the estimated total power in the posteriorly located IOL and 1/3 anteriorly based in the assumption that should IOL decentration appear, the anteriorly lower-powered IOL will induce less visual consequences to the patient. The surgeon should systematically monitor power errors to arrive at an appropriate adjustment to the formula-predicted value. This will vary by formula, and by surgeon. Make sure that appropriate constants are used. In secondary cases (underpowered pseudophakes), the necessary additional power is provided by implanting a second IOL of appropriate power with haptics fixated in the sulcus. In secondary cases the refraction is used to determine the power requirement. Our lens choices, strategies, and power formulas for secondary cases are presented in Table 3–3. We use PMMA three-piece biconvex IOLs with an optic size of 5.5 mm for primary piggy-back cases. The PMMA optic is thinner than a silicone optic making bag-fixation of 2 IOLs easier (Fig. 3–4). The material is more firm so the IOL

TABLE 3–3. Recommended IOL Styles and Power Calculation Methods When Using Piggy-back IOLs for High Hyperopes and Residual Refractive Error

I. Primary Piggy-backs (High Hyperopes)
  A. Formula: Holladay 2
    • Total required power is divided in half between two lenses
    • Both IOLs are placed in the bag
    • Haptics are aligned
  B. Lenses:
    • Ioptex UPB320GS
      PMMA, biconvex, 5.5 mm optic, one-piece IOL
      A Constant: 117.9
      Diopter range: 16.0 to 24.0
    • Storz P359UV
      PMMA, equiconvex, 5.5 mm optic, one-piece IOL
      A Constant: 118.0
      Diopter Range: 4.0 to 34.0
II. Secondary Piggy-backs
  A. Formula: Underpowered Pseudophake (hyperope)
    1. Short eye (<21 mm):   P = (1.5 × sph. equ.) +1
    2. Avg. eye (22–26 mm):   P = (1.4 × sph. equ.) +1
    3. Long eye (>27 mm):   P = (1.3 × sph. equ.) +1
  B. Lenses:
    • Storz PO47UV
      PMMA, equiconvex, 6.0 mm optic, sulcus, one-piece IOL
      A Constant: 118.0
      Diopter Range: 4.0 to 30.0
    • Allergan AMO PS60AMB
      PMMA, concave/convex, 6.0 mm optic, sulcus, one-piece IOL
      A Constant: 116.7
      Diopter Range: 1.0 to 5.0
  C. Formula: Overpowered Pseudophake
    1. Short eye (<21 mm):   P = (1.5 × sph. equ.) -1
    2. Avg. eye (22–26 mm):   P = (1.4 × sph. equ.) -1
    3. Long eye (>27 mm):   P = (1.3 × sph. equ.) -1
  D. Lenses:
    • Allergan AMO PS60AZB
      PMMA, Concave/convex, 6.0 mm optic, one-piece, post chamber IOL
      A Constant 116.0
      Diopter range: −1.0 to −10.0
NOTE: A Constants: Not necessary to consider for Secondary IOLs
  • Secondary IOLs are very low powers
  • IOLs are always in the same position (sulcus)

will hold position better. As stated, we generally use a self-sealing scleral tunnel incision in these cases. The incision length must accommodate the 5.5 mm optic and a 5.5 mm clear corneal incision would have an increased risk of infection. The incision is placed in the steep meridian to correct preexisting astigmatism. In some cases limbal or corneal relaxing incisions are also performed to correct a preexisting astigmatism.[15] Both IOLs are bag-fixated with the haptics aligned (Fig. 3–5). The postsurgical medication regimen is detailed in Table 3–2.

We perform an immediate postoperative refraction to detect any power "surprises" which may then be corrected by an immediate exchange of the anterior lens.

Surgical Management of the Shallow Anterior Chamber

Shallow anterior chambers are something we've grown to respect. When the axial length is less than 20.5 mm there is certainly a difference in difficulty both with the incision and with phacoemulsification. Clear corneal incisions (CCIs) are more difficult because they are large in proportion to the corneal diameter so we often employ a scleral tunnel in these cases. Although CCIs are possible, there

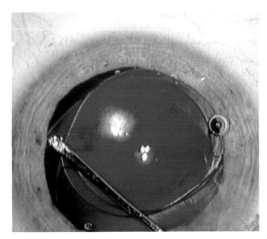

FIGURE 3–4. Rotating the anterior piggy-back lens into the capsular bag.

is likely to be extended corneal edema in small eyes. The anatomy of an eye 18.5 mm or less makes surgery more difficult and definitely precludes the use of a CCI.

In very short eyes, when we insert the phaco tip, the iris may prolapse up to the cornea if the corneal lip is not far enough anteriorly. When this occurs we inject Viscoat into the mouth of the incision. This enables the phaco tip to be more easily inserted into the anterior segment. Sometimes it may be difficult to

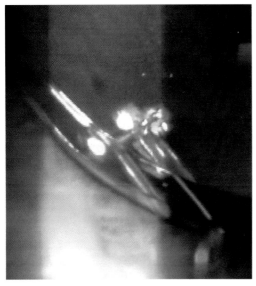

FIGURE 3–5. Bag-fixated IOLs with the haptics aligned (Photo provided by Dr. L. W. Lu).

form the anterior chamber if the eye is hard. In this case it's best to massage the eye to avoid dealing with a too shallow anterior chamber and compromised working conditions which may result in corneal edema or vitreous loss.

With short eyes there is a higher risk of pupillary block while the pupil is dilated. This can result in a hard eye making phaco difficult. Another problem with microphthalmic eyes is that of choroidal effusion or fluid misdirection which can increase the pressure in the eye. Fortunately, with a self-sealing incision, the procedure may be easily stopped for several hours or a day pressure comes down. We encourage surgeons not to feel that surgery must be completed on the same day if the eye becomes hard. This is my general practice. There are alternatives to delaying or postponing surgery that also work. Many surgeons prefer a pars plana tap removing vitreous. A block may be used with a super Pinky, Honnan balloon, or another device to lower the IOP. If these alternatives don't work it's best to stop surgery and resume another day when pressure is lower. There is *no medical disadvantage in waiting and coming back*. This is a very important concept when dealing with a small eye.

Titrating the Postoperative Refraction

Following appropriate IOL power selection and good surgical technique, patients achieve excellent visual results. If the anterior-most IOL is misplaced, power errors can occur. For example if it is completely in the sulcus there will be a 3 to 6 D shift in the myopic direction. In one instance, a front IOL tilted, with one haptic in the bag and the other in the sulcus. This can result in both a shift in refraction in the myopic direction and induced refractive astigmatism. Even if there is no misplacement of the IOL, with current formulas there are still power "surprises" in some cases. When topical anesthesia is used, the patient can actually be refracted on the same or next day to determine if there is a power error. An immediate exchange of the anterior-most IOL can be performed in a very low-risk, nontraumatic procedure. In this way, the refraction may be titrated appropriately and all patients will enjoy good refractive outcome.

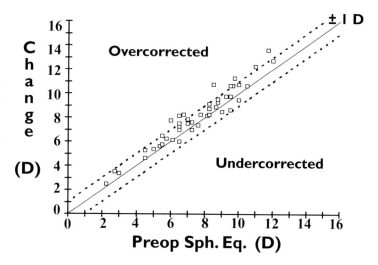

FIGURE 3–6. (Gills) Scatterplot of achieved refractive change in spherical equivalent versus the preoperative spherical equivalent in 51 eyes with short axial lengths which received double implants. Most eyes were targeted for a residual refractive error of -0.5 D, although a few cases were targeted for 1.0–2.0 D of myopia for monovision. The targeted and achieved changes in spherical equivalent are highly correlated.

■ Results of Piggy-Back IOLs in High Hyperopes

Earlier we reported the results of eight bilateral highly hyperopic patients (16 eyes) who received two or three implants in each eye to provide adequate power.[10] In that series, 75% of cases were within a diopter of emmetropia and the rest were mildly (1 to 2 D) myopic. Visual results were good. In that study we also evaluated a larger group of underpowered pseudophakes who received a second IOL to provide the additional power needed. These cases received primary double implants in the contralateral eye. Ninety-two percent of the eyes with secondary double implants were within a diopter of emmetropia. One other finding of that study was that among our primary double implant cases, 60% of the eyes had an increased depth of focus; that is, they had uncorrected near vision of J1-J3 while still maintaining good uncorrected distance acuity (20/40 or better) at near-emmetropic refractions.

The results of a more recent series of 51 highly hyperopic cataract patients are summarized in Figures 3–6 and 3–7. Mean preoperative hyperopia was 7.38 D (standard error = 0.34, range of 2.25 to 12 D). Total required power ranged from 30 to 55 D. Mean postoperative spherical equivalent was 0.56 D (standard error = 0.09, range of −2.25 to 0.87 D). Figure 3–6 is a scatterplot of the change in spherical equivalent versus the preoperative refraction. Eighty-two percent of cases were within a diopter of emmetropia and 53% were within 0.5 D (Figure 3–7). Most of the cases had been targeted for a refraction of −0.5 D. A few were targeted for 1 to 1.5 D of myopia for monovision. Nine of the 51 cases (17%) were amblyopic or had conditions affecting visual outcome. In 16 of the 51 eyes, relaxing incisions were performed to correct preexisting astigmatism. The reduction in cylinder for these cases averaged about a diopter.

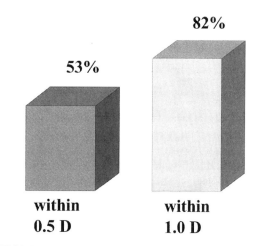

FIGURE 3–7. (Gills) Bar chart illustrating the deviation from emmetropia among the 51 eyes studied. Fifty-three percent were within 0.5 D of emmetropia and 82% were within a diopter of emmetropia.

■ Future Concepts

For too long highly hyperopic patients have been at a disadvantage as they approached cataract surgery. They have had to settle for less than optimal visual and refractive outcomes. The innovative approach of implanting piggy-back IOLs to provide adequate power has made a world of difference to the hyperopic patient. This strategy has been very successful and has provided a strong impetus to improve power calculation methods for short eyes. Now that we know we can *provide* enough power using double implants, we can no longer countenance less accurate power calculation methods for short axial lengths. In the near future we can expect power calculation to be much better. Indeed, we see greatly improved predictions in the early testing of the Holladay 2 formula, which uses more measurements to accurately determine power in short eyes and which factors in power adjustments when two IOLs are implanted.[1]

Another aid to providing better power prediction will be a better estimate of the exact position of the IOL in the eye. In this regard, an important additional measurement to obtain would be the position of the ciliary sulcus. It is known that the IOL with flat loops centers about 0.2 mm behind the center of the sulcus. It has not been possible to measure the location of the ciliary sulcus in the past. With newer ultrasound units we can measure the distance from the front of the cornea to the ciliary sulcus. These units are generally used for other diagnostic work but will probably be adapted for use in measuring the sulcus location to provide an accurate measurement of the IOL location. When this occurs, we can look forward to even fewer power "surprises" in the high hyperope.

Also in the future will be the ability to piggy-back toric and spherical IOLs to correct high levels of astigmatism along with high hyperopia. This will be an improvement in the management of astigmatism for patients with high cylinder.

As occurs with all new IOL technology and new surgical technique, new insertion technology will follow. A special piggy-back lens holder will be an important addition.

Both patient and surgeon will derive great satisfaction as all these goals are achieved.

■ Tips and Pearls for Managing High Hyperopes:

1. Careful Measurement of the Axial Length.

While this is important for every patient, it can't be stressed enough when working with the high hyperope. A small measurement error is a much larger percentage of the axial length in a short eye and therefore more significant for the postoperative refraction. We recommend immersion ultrasound for the most accurate and reproducible results.

2. Measure Additional Parameters of the Anterior Segment.

It is critical to measure the corneal diameter, lens thickness and anterior chamber depth to determine if the anterior segment is disproportionate to the length of the eye. Holladay's IOL Consultant software takes these additional factors into consideration for a more accurate result.

3. Beware of the Shallow A/C.

Consider using a peribulbar block with pressure to deepen the A/C. Proceed with caution and deepen the anterior chamber as needed with viscoelastic.

4. Watch for Choroidal Effusion.

This problem is particularly common in the extremely hyperopic eye, especially in cases of microphthalmos.

5. Discuss the Target Refraction with the Patient.

Hyperopes are generally good candidates for monovision. Consider targeting the first eye for near to intermediate vision.

6. Check the Postoperative Refraction Immediately After Surgery.

If the refraction isn't as anticipated, consider exchanging the IOL immediately.

7. Consider Making a Scleral Cataract Incision Rather Than a Clear Corneal Incision.

This not only provides more room to work, there is less corneal edema and involvement.

REFERENCES

1. Holladay JR. Achieving emmetropia in extremely short eyes. Presented at the 1996 Annual Meeting of the American Academy of Ophthalmology Chicago, IL; 1996.
2. Sanders DR, Retzlaff JA, Kraff MC. A-scan biometry and IOL implant power calculations. In: Focal Points: Clinical Modules for Ophthalmologists. San Francisco, CA: American Academy of Ophthalmology 1995;10:1–14.
3. Holladay JT, Prager TC, Chandler TY, et al. A three-part system for refining intraocular lens power calculation. J Cataract Refract Surg 1988;14:17–24.
4. Retzlaff JA, Sanders DR, Kraff MC. Lens Implant Power Calculation: A Manual for Ophthalmologists and Biometrists, 3rd ed. Thorofore, NJ: Slack; 1990.
5. Sanders DR, Retzlaff JA, Kraff MC, et al. Comparison of the SRK/T formula and other theoretical and regression formulas. J Cataract Refract Surg 1990;16:341–346.
6. Hoffer KJ. The Hoffer Q formula. A comparison of theoretic and regression formulas. J Cataract Refract Surg 1993;19:700–712.
7. Holladay JT, Gills JP, Leidlein JL, Cherchio M. Achieving emmetropia in extremely short eyes with two piggyback posterior chamber intraocular lenses. Ophthalmology 1996;103:1118–1123.
8. Smith WJ. Modern Optical Emmetropia. The Design of Optical Systems. NY: McGraw-Hill; 1966;50–52.
9. Gayton JL, Sanders VN. Implanting two posterior chamber intraocular lenses in a case of microphthalmos. J Cataract Refract Surg 1993;19:776–777.
10. Gills JP. The implantation of multiple intraocular lenses to optimize visual results in hyperopic cataract patients and under-powered pseudophakes. Best Papers of Sessions, 1995 Symposium on Cataract IOL and Refractive Surgery Special Issue, 1996.
11. Gayton JL, Raanan MG. Reducing refractive error in high hyperopes with double implants. In: Gayton JL (ed). Maximizing Results. Thorofare, NJ: Slack; 1996; 139–148.
12. Holladay JT, Prager TC, Ruiz RS, Lewis JW. Improving the predictability of intraocular lens power calculations. Arch Ophthalmol 1986;104:539–541.
13. Shammus HJF. A comparison of immersion and contact techniques for axial length measurement. Am Intraocular Implant Soc J 1984;10:444.
14. Gills JP, Cherchio M, Raanan MG. The use of intraoperative unpreserved lidocaine to control discomfort during IOL surgery under topical anesthesia. J Cataract Refract Surg 1997;23:545–550.
15. Gills JP, Cherchio M. Relaxing incisions for correcting astigmatism and optimizing near and distance vision. Presented at the 1995 annual meeting of the American Academy of Ophthalmology.

4

Phacoemulsification in Patients with High Astigmatism

LUIS W. LU AND STEPHEN HOLLIS

The surgical management of astigmatism in patients presenting with cataracts has been a controversial subject, and no one technique or management plan has been accepted by the ophthalmologic community in general. We will discuss management issues and procedures in combined surgery for cataracts and astigmatism.

The goal of surgical management of astigmatism is to obtain the best possible vision without the use of corrective lenses after small incision cataract surgery. This is obtained by affecting the spherical component and the astigmatic component of the refractive error. To correct the spherical component, the ophthalmologist must use an implant with precisely the correct power. In addition, the ophthalmologist must reduce the astigmatism without overcorrecting the patient or changing the axis.

In refractive surgery we correct the refractive astigmatism, but when done simultaneously with cataract surgery it is best to operate on topography astigmatism. The lenticular component will be gone after the cataract is removed, so the corneal astigmatism should yield the accurate reading.

■ Considerations

Correcting the Spherical Component

The third generation formulas have been the best way to calculate the power of the intraocular lens (IOL). The SRK/T was apparently the best formula for patients with myopia and an axial length of more than 26.0 mm; the third generation Holladay 1 formula for eyes with an axial length between 24.5 and 26.0 mm. The Hoffer Q was preferred for eyes with an axial length of less than 22.0 mm, and the average of the three of them was the preferred formula for eyes with axial length between 22.0 and 24.5 mm.

At the present time, calculations on patients with axial lengths between 22 and 25 mm with corneal powers between 42 and 46 D will do well with current third generation formulas. In cases outside this range, the Holladay 2 should be used to assure accuracy.

When the surgeon is calculating the IOL power, he must also take into account the amount of astigmatism that needs to be corrected if transverse incisions are planned. The two main formulas are the Maloney and Nordan's in which 20 to 25% of the power of the astigmatism to be corrected is added to the IOL power calculation (i.e., if a patient is calculated to receive a 21.0 D IOL and have 2.0 D of astigmatism corrected, 0.5D will be added to the 21.0 D and the final needed power will be 21.5 D).

When using the Arcuate Incision or the Hollis Limbal Relaxing Incision method no power is added to the calculated IOL power.

Correcting the Astigmatic Component

About 5% of patients who come for cataract surgery have a minimal amount of keratometric astigmatism of less than 0.5 D. About 75% have less than 1.25 D. Three to five percent of patients have an oblique astigmatism. About 60% have against-the-rule (ATR) astigmatism, and 30% with-the-rule (WTR). The statistics are influenced by the fact that patients who come for cataract surgery have an average age of 70 years.[1]

The suggested corrections below, are designed to be used with temporal clear-corneal incisions, unless specified otherwise.

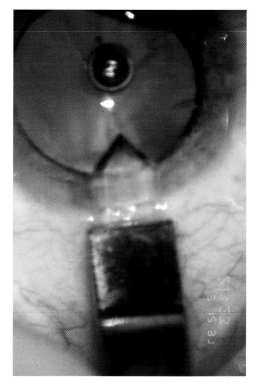

FIGURE 4–1. Stab, single-plane CCI.

Patients with Minimal Astigmatism

This first category includes those patients (5%) with minimum amount of *with-the-rule or against-the-rule astigmatism of less than 0.5 D*. These patients need to have a cataract incision that will induce a minimum amount of astigmatism or no astigmatism at all. In theses cases, the surgeon should try to match the postoperative corneal curvature with the preoperative curvature.

A single-plane, very peripheral temporal stab incision is used (Fig. 4–1). An incision of this type, should induce between 0 to 0.50 D, and usually no more than a 0.37 D of induced with-the-rule astigmatism,[2] preferably using the 3-D diamond blade for incisions of 3.0, 2.8, or 2.5 mm. After the IOL insertion a 3.0 to a 3.2 mm incision will be obtained.

Patients with Mild Astigmatism

The second group of patients includes those who have more than 0.5 D but less than 1.25 D of astigmatism. The patients, who comprise 75% of cases, need a cataract incision that will decrease the preoperative astigmatism.

For patients with 0.5 to 1.25 D of ATR astigmatism, a two-step grooved incision is indicated. The grove depth varies from 300 to 600 μ. The deeper the groove, the greater the effect, and up to 0.75 D of astigmatism correction may be accomplished (Fig. 4–2). Age is also a factor, the older the patient, the greater the effect. If about 1.25 D of cylindrical correction is to be obtained, a Limbal Relaxing Incision (LRI) can be combined with a single-plane cataract incision, with the LRI of 6 mm affecting 1.0 D.[3]

For patients with 0.5 to 1.25 D of WTR astigmatism, the astigmatically neutral, single-plane, ungrooved clear corneal incision is used and the corneal relaxing incision (CRI) or LRI is placed on-axis, if needed. In cases of oblique astigmatism (between 30–60 degrees or 120–150 axis), the same ungrooved incision is indicated, with the addition of a CRI or LRI at the appropriate axis, if required.

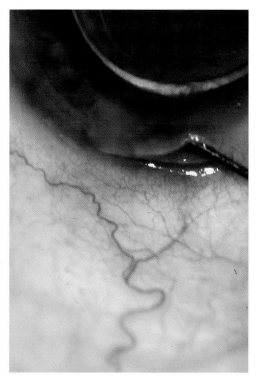

FIGURE 4–2. Grooved two-step CCI.

The surgeon may elect to use on-axis cataract surgery incision for these patients using a short scleral tunnel, starting 1 mm posterior to the limbus and extending the incision to 1.75 mm into clear cornea for patients in this category. A 3.5 to 4.0 mm incision should correct about 0.5 D, a 5.0 mm incision about 0.75 D, and a 6.0 mm about 1.00 D. We prefer not to perform unsutured clear cornea wounds obliquely or superiorly since have demonstrated higher degrees of corneal endothelial cell loss (Hoffer & Grabow).

The amount of astigmatism to be affected depends also of the patient's age, in a 50 to 60-year-old we prefer to leave the patient with a WTR astigmatism of about 1 D, while in a 70-year-old patient, close to astigmatically neutral. The decision should also include the astigmatic status of the opposite eye and if surgery is foreseen to be required in the future. Therefore, over-correction of ATR and under-correction of WTR is not always recommended.

Patients with Moderate (1.5 to 3.0 D) and High (more than 3.00 D) Astigmatism

This third group of patients are the 10 to 20% with an astigmatism higher than 1.25 D.

For moderate degrees of ATR astigmatism of 1.50 to 3.0 D, the two-step grooved incision is used. For this amount of correction needed, the surgeon will have several options:

1. Moving the vertical groove centrally 0.5 to 1.0 mm reducing the optical zone (OZ) of the two-step cataract incision.[2]

2. Keratolenticuloplasty:
   For 1.50 D   Incision of 3.00 mm OZ 9
        2.00 D   2.50 mm OZ 8 and a CRI of 2.5 mm OZ 8
        2.50 D   2.50 mm OZ 9 and a CRI of 2.5 mm OZ 7
        3.00 D   3.00 mm OZ 9 and a CRI of 3.0 mm OZ 7

   CRIs are made at 100% depth of pachometry at the area of the incision.[4]

3. A Modified Lindstrom Nomogram:
   A two-step grooved incision at OZ 10 with the addition of:
   For 1.50 D   2.5 mm transverse   at OZ 7
        2.00 D   2.5 mm arcuate   at OZ 7 (45*)
        3.00 D   3.0 mm arcuate   at OZ 7 (60*)
   at a depth of 600 μ.[5]

4. The use of Limbal Relaxing Incisions: A 6.0 mm in cord length incision is required for each diopter of correction up to 2 D at a 600 μ blade depth.[3]
   For 1.0 D   (1) LRI of 6.0 mm (at the side away from the cataract incision).
        2.0 D   (2) LRI's of 6 mm
        3.0 D   (2) LRI's of 8 mm

5. The use of the Toric IOL, soon available with the 2.00 and 3.50 D models (STAAR) for approximately 1.00 to 1.25 D and 2.00 to 2.5 D of cylinder, respectively.

Again, the two-step grooved incision has an age related effect, as well as the CRIs, producing in certain cases an unstable refraction of up to 2 to 3 months in the elderly. LRIs are a weaker corrective procedure; however, they produce less postoperative glare, less discomfort, and the incisions heal faster. Unlike CRIs, making the incision at the limbus preserves the optical qualities of the cornea. LRIs are a more forgiving procedure and significant overcorrections are rare.

The astigmatic correction can be performed just before the cataract surgery, at the end of the procedure, or as a second surgery. With the improved predictability of the AK procedures, we prefer to make all the astigmatic corrective incisions first before entering the eye through the cataract incision, as the eye is more firm and the incision depths are more reliable.

If corneal topography shows the symmetrical bow tie type of corneal mapping, the correction will require about equal, symmetrical on-axis incisions. If it differs (i.e., from the nasal to the temporal part), the choice depends upon the location of the main amount of astigmatism. Inferior arcuate incisions are the more unstable.

For moderate degrees of WTR astigmatism of 1.5 to 3.0 D, the surgeon again will have several different options depending of the approach preferred for the cataract surgery:

1. If temporal clear corneal incision (CCI) is the choice, the astigmatically almost neutral, single-plane, ungrooved CCI is used, and the appropriate AK-CRI incisions are placed on-axis (A Modified Lindstrom Nomogram on the steep vertical axis).
   LRIs can also be used on the steep axis (Fig. 4–3).
2. If a short sclero-corneal tunnel incision is decided, part of the astigmatism will be corrected by the 4 to 6 mm incision itself, with the addition of an AK for the remaining astigmatism to be corrected, i.e., if 3.00 D is to be corrected, a 5 mm, short tunnel incision should correct 0.75 D of the astigmatism, the remaining 2.25 D can be treated with a single 45 degrees arcuate incision at OZ 7.

Astigmatism higher than 4.0 D will certainly require additional AK incisions. For 4.00 D two arcuate incisions of 2.50 mm at OZ 7

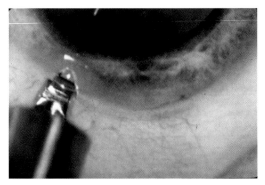

FIGURE 4–3. Limbal relaxing incision previous to CCI.

(45*) depth of 600 μ. For 6.00 D of astigmatism, a triple set of incisions may be desired, especially in the younger patient, at optical zones of 6.0, 7.0, and 8.0.[2]

In patients with high astigmatism, further astigmatic surgery might be required if again further correction is considered necessary. This can be accomplished redeepening the AK incisions with additional AK incisions or with the use of excimer laser. Arcuate incisions in the elderly can induce a substantial amount of overcorrection.

■ Surgical Procedure

The preoperative cataract surgery evaluation includes the manual and automated keratometric readings, as well as the corneal topography. The type of surgical incision is planned and the topographic mapping is taken to the operating room and is used to pinpoint the exact location of the astigmatism. The axis of the astigmatism is marked with a sterile marking pen.

A single-plane CCI is performed for minimal astigmatism corrections. After asking the patient to look at the microscope's light, the peripheral temporal stab incision is performed with the 3-D diamond blade while fixating the eye either using the index finger or a fixation ring (Fig. 4–4).

When a 300 μ groove is required for the two-step grooved incision, the Beaver guarded knife or the 15 degree diamond blade is uti-

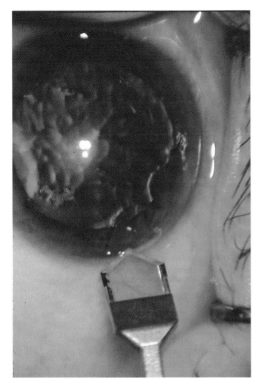

FIGURE 4–4. Fixating the eye.

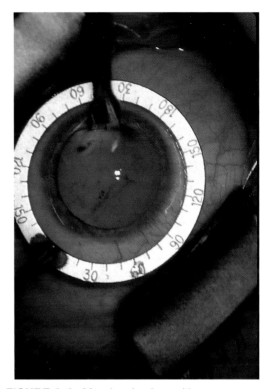

FIGURE 4–6. Mendez ring in position.

lized. The same diamond blade can be used when a 400 μ(Williamson) or a 500 to 600 μ groove (Langerman) is needed.

Should an AK be needed, the 7.0 or 8.0 mm Hoffer optical zone corneal marker is used with gentle pressure over the cornea (Fig. 4–5), since the epithelium may loosen after the use of topical anesthesia. The Mendez corneal ring is applied (Fig. 4–6). The

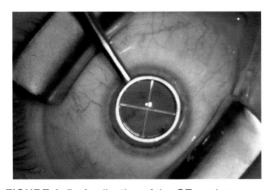

FIGURE 4–5. Application of the OZ marker.

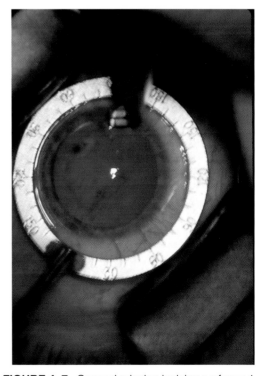

FIGURE 4–7. Corneal relaxing incision performed.

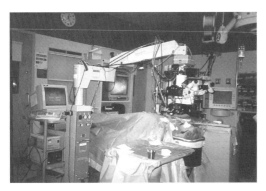

FIGURE 4–8. PAR system.

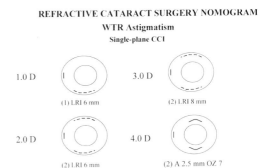

FIGURE 4–9. Nomogram for WTR astigmatism.

Grandon T marker is used for transverse incisions, the Lindstrom corneal marker for the arcuate incisions and, when LRI is needed, the 6 mm cord length is marked with a Castroviejo caliper while keeping the Mendez ring in position. The incision is then performed (Fig. 4–7).

The type, length, and location of the AK incision is predetermined. The astigmatic correction is qualitatively calculated using the Maloney or Karickhoff keratoscope, and when a real-time quantitative measurement is required for patients with moderate to high astigmatism, intraoperative topography is done with the PAR Visual System (Fig. 4–8). This is obtained by increasing the microscope magnification to 1.8 and applying a drop of diluted fluorescein on the cornea. Alignment is done on the background grid observed. After the image is captured, BSS solution is used to wash out the fluorescein stain.

■ Tips and Pearls

1. For patients with minimal amount of astigmatism (<0.5 D), a single-plane, very peripheral stab clear corneal incision is recommended. The same is indicated for patients with WTR astigmatism of less than 1.25 D (Fig. 4–9).
2. For patients with mild ATR astigmatism (between 0.5 and 1.25 D), a two-step grooved incision is suggested, keeping in mind that the deeper the groove the more correction obtained (Fig. 4–10).
3. In patients with moderate (1.5 to 3.0 D) and high (>3.0 D) astigmatism the following nomogram is suggested when combined with Temporal Clear Corneal Cataract Incision: Table 4–1.
4. Some advantages of the LRIs is that the procedure is almost pain-free, more forgiving about the exact axis of the astigmatism, and that overcorrections are rare. In general, when combined with cataract surgery a 6 mm cord length LRI will correct 1.0 D of astigmatism; two 6 mm cord length LRI will correct 2.0 D of astigmatism, and two 8 mm cord length LRI will correct 3.0 D of astigmatism.

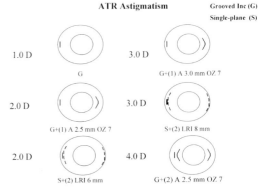

FIGURE 4–10. Nomogram for ATR astigmatism.

Table 4–1. WTR and ATR Astigmatism Correction in T–CCI Cataract Surgery

	Diopters		Incision	AK (at steep axis)		
				CRI	or	LRI
WTR	<0.5	D	Single-plane(S)	No		No
	0.5–1.25	D	Single-plane	No		No
	1.5	D	Single-plane	1 (T) 2.5 mm OZ 7	or	(1) 6 mm cord at 90°
	2.0	D	Single-plane	1 (A) 2.5 mm OZ 7	or	(2) 6 mm cord at 90°
	3.0	D	Single-plane	1 (A) 3.0 mm OZ 7	or	(2) 8 mm cord at 90°
	4.0	D	Single-plane	2 (A) 2.5 mm OZ 7		
ATR	<0.50	D	Single-plane	No		No
	0.5–1.25	D	Grooved (G)	No		No
	1.5	D	G OZ 9		or	S + (1) 6 mm cord at 180°
	2.0	D	G OZ 10	+ 1 (A) 2.5 mm OZ 7	or	S + (2) 6 mm cord at 180°
	3.0	D	G OZ 10	+ 1 (A) 3.0 mm OZ 7	or	S + (2) 8 mm cord at 180°
	4.0	D	G OZ 9	+ 2 (A) 2.5 mm OZ 7		

Depth: 100% of pachometry at the area of planned CRI or 600 μ if pachometry not available.
600 μ for LRI

REFERENCES

1. Lu LW, Contreras C. Incidence of Astigmatism in the cataract population. XIX PanAmerican Congress of Ophthalmology. July 1993. Caracas, Venezuela.
2. Grabow HB. Six Steps to Sphericity: An Astigmatism management System for Temporal, Clear-Corneal, Cataract Surgery. ACES 1997. Ft. Lauderdale, FL.
3. Gills, J. Limbal Relaxing Incisions. ASCRS meeting 1996. Seattle, WA.
4. Kershner, RM. Refractive Keratotomy for Cataract Surgery and the Correction of Astigmatism. Thorofare, NJ: Slack, Inc.; 1994.
5. Lu LW. Surgical Management of Astigmatism. Highlights of Ophthalmology. In press.

5

Phacoemulsification in Patients with Fuchs' Corneal Dystrophy

GAVIN G. BAHADUR, JACK M. DODICK, AND RICHARD P. GIBRALTER

Fuchs' dystrophy is an asymmetric bilateral disorder of the cornea characterized by abnormal endothelial cells which can lead to corneal clouding and poor visual acuity. This entity is more commonly observed in women over 40 and is usually inherited in an autosomal dominant fashion with variable penetrance. The edema usually begins centrally and moves to the periphery over time. Examination characteristically reveals corneal thickening and cornea guttata (Fig. 5–1).[1,2] In severe cases, the corneal surface may become irregular due to bullous changes (Fig. 5–2). The progression of the disease varies but may be aggravated by intraocular surgery. When cataract surgery is performed, special care should be taken to protect the corneal endothelium from unnecessary manipulations.

■ Preoperative Evaluation

Complete eye examination, keratometry, and A-scans are performed as with all patients undergoing cataract surgery. Careful slit lamp examination is used to determine whether there is sufficient corneal edema to warrant a triple procedure (cataract extraction, IOL implantation, and PK) (Figs. 5–3 and 5–4). We believe that neither endothelial cell count nor corneal pachymetry is reliable predictor of subsequent corneal decompensation. Consequently, we do not use specific cutoff values for endothelial cell density nor corneal thickness in guiding our management.

■ Combined Procedure vs. Sequential Surgery

If a patient with Fuchs' dystrophy has a visually significant cataract, we carefully evaluate the status of the cornea in order to determine whether to perform cataract extraction alone or in conjunction with a penetrating keratoplasty.

For patients with symptomatic visual compromise which is due to *both* lenticular opacification and corneal clouding, we plan a triple procedure: penetrating keratoplasty (PK), standard extracapsular cataract extraction, and intraocular lens (IOL) implantation to achieve visual rehabilitation (Fig. 5–5). Performing PK followed by cataract surgery in this setting unnecessarily increases costs and recovery time, and also subjects the patient to a second operation.

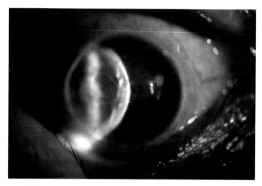

FIGURE 5–1. Corneal thickening and cornea guttata.

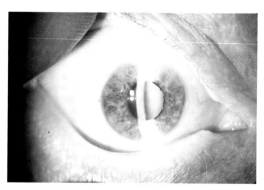

FIGURE 5–3. Slit lamp examination.

A retrospective review by Peneros et al. performed at Wills Eye Hospital compared the results of patients who underwent PK, standard ECCE, and PCIOL implantation (triple procedure) with those who underwent PK alone followed by standard ECCE or phacoemulsification with IOL implantation. This study concluded that there were no statistically significant differences between the two groups in best-corrected visual acuity, refractive errors (including severity of astigmatism), and graft clarity.[3]

When performing a triple procedure (cataract extraction, IOL implantation, and PK), we prefer an "open sky" extracapsular cataract extraction in which I/A of cortical remnants is carried out manually using a blunt 30 gauge cannula and 3 cc syringe. The greatest advantage of cataract removal by phacoemulsification is the reduction of incision size. In a triple procedure, the PK negates any potential advantages related to cataract incision size and consequently, phacoemulsification has no distinct advantage in this setting.

Malbran has presented an interesting two-step procedure in which only the corneal epithelium is removed first, so that phacoemulsification and IOL implantation can occur in a closed system. The PK is then performed after IOL implantation.[4] In our experience, the "open-sky" approach has been well tolerated and we have not perceived a need to move to a closed system method.

Wen we opt to perform phacoemulsification with IOL alone in a patient with Fuchs' dystrophy, we have a thorough discussion of the risks of subsequent corneal decompensation and the potential need for penetrating keratoplasty in the future. Any strong feelings the patient may have concerning the number of operations required are taken into consideration.

In cases where it is unclear whether or not a combined procedure is needed, the patient is informed of the options and engaged in a dis-

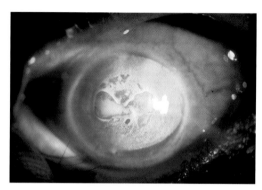

FIGURE 5–2. Bullous keratopathy.

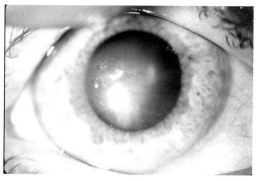

FIGURE 5–4. Cataract in the presence of Fuchs' Corneal Dystrophy.

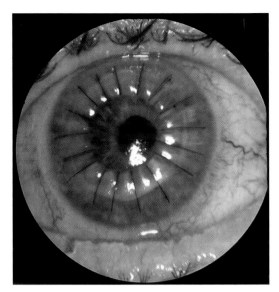

FIGURE 5-5. Immediately after triple procedure (photo provided by Dr. Lu).

cussion concerning the total number of operations, recovery time, anesthesia risks, and costs. A joint decision between the surgeon and patient can be made regarding the best approach for these cases.

■ Phacoemulsification Modifications in Fuchs' Dystrophy:

Choice of Intraocular Lens

Polymethylmethacrylate (PMMA) lenses are biologically inert and well-suited for the Fuchs' patient. Recently, we have used acrylic foldable lenses exclusively as these appear to be well-tolerated and may have a decreased incidence of posterior capsular opacification. Silicone foldable implants are not recommended due to a potential for increased inflammation, incompatibility with silicone oil procedures, and pitting during YAG laser capsulotomy.

Surgical Procedure: Phacoemulsification with IOL

We routinely perform phacoemulsification procedures with topical and intracameral anesthesia. Diazepam (10 mg) is given to the patient orally 30 minutes prior to surgery. Topical proparacaine (0.5%) is administered to the operative eye three times, every 10 minutes. After entering the anterior chamber, we inject 0.3 to 0.5 cc of 1% lidocaine PF (Methyl Paraben Free) into the anterior chamber. Periodically during the case, 1 mg of intravenous diazepam is administered as needed for patient comfort.

No retrobulbar nor peribulbar injections are used, eliminating the serious risks of globe penetration and retrobulbar hemorrhage. The risks of anesthetic injection into the extraocular muscles or optic nerve sheath are also eliminated. Furthermore, no additional fluid volume is added to the orbit, preventing extrinsic positive pressure on the globe.

We make a 3.0 mm clear corneal incision with a diamond blade rather than a stainless steel keratome to create a fairly atraumatic entry with minimal tissue distortion and smooth wound edges which form a watertight seal and cause minimal slippage against the rule (usually 0.5–0.75 D).

Creating the incision in the cornea rather than the sclera also obviates the need for conjunctival manipulation, eliminates the tissue distortion caused by electrocautery, and also preserves normal limbal architecture avoiding postoperative tear film abnormalities which could aggravate any subsequent bullous corneal changes in the future.

We use an adhesive rather than strongly cohesive viscoelastic of low to moderate molecular weight in order to protect the corneal endothelium. The viscoelastic is injected into the anterior chamber periodically throughout the case, particularly during nuclear rotation, cracking, or chopping to maintain its protective effects on the endothelium.

Special care is taken to avoid contact between the endothelium and all intraocular instruments. Similarly, the surgeon must pay particular attention to Descemet's membrane during the insertion of instruments through the wound, to avoid creating a Descemet's detachment. If stripping of Descemet's membrane occurs, it should be gently replaced in its original position and tamponaded with viscoelastic, air, or sulfur hexafluoride gas (SF_6). Large detachments rarely require suturing.

Several nucleofractis techniques may be used to minimize the amount of ultrasound power administered to ocular structures. In our technique, two identical phaco choppers are used along with the Alcon Legacy Series 200000 phacoemulsification unit with the Kelman microtip. Use of the Kelman microtip may allow for greater efficiency and can decrease total energy required.

We recommend chopping the nucleus into four or more fragments without the use of ultrasound energy. We employ a technique of chopping originally described by Jochen Kammenn of Dortmund, Germany, which offers significant advantages over many other commonly used methods of nucleofactis.

In this technique, the nucleus is fragmented into four or more pieces without the use of ultrasound power, greatly reducing the total amount of energy administered to the anterior chamber, making the procedure well-suited for a patient with Fuchs' endothelial dystrophy.

We use two identical phaco choppers. Each chopping instrument must be a minimum of 1.5 mm in length (preferably 2.0 mm) at its distal 90-degree bend, as shown (Fig. 5–6). The tips of the instruments should be spherical and finely polished so as to be atraumatic to the lens capsule.

After performing a capsulorhexis at least 5.0 mm in diameter, the phacoemulsification handpiece of the Legacy 20,000 with the straight microtip is used to aspirate anterior lens cortex with vacuum settings of 400 mmHg, using no phaco power.

Next, the two choppers are inserted at 90 degree angles: one through the principal incision at 11:00 and the second through a clear corneal paracentesis at 2:00. The instruments are inserted nearly parallel to the iris, between the anterior capsule and the lens. Each chopper is gently rotated and positioned so that the blunt end faces the posterior capsule at the equatorial region of the lens (Fig. 5–6-A).

In a smooth controlled motion, the two choppers are drawn together toward the visual axis, thereby chopping the lens in half (Fig. 5–6-B). Next, the choppers are positioned on either side of the inferior heminucleus (at 5:00 and centrally, Fig. 5–6-C) and are carefully drawn together, creating two distinct quadrants (Fig. 5–6-D). The choppers are then placed at 11:00 and centrally, and the superior heminucleus is fractured into two quadrants, as shown (Figs. 5–6-E and 5–6-F).

Once quartered, the nuclear fragments are removed using vacuum settings of 300 to 400 mmHg and aspiration flow rates of 30 to 35 cc/min. During phacoemulsification of the nuclear quadrants, a Sinskey Hook may be used to facilitate bringing nuclear fragments into the phaco tip. Using this technique, we have emulsified a nucleus of moderate density (up to 3+ nuclear sclerosis), using an average of 10% phaco power over a total of 1 to 2 minutes. These power and time parameters are a significant reduction from those routinely required in our cases in which we use phacoemulsification to groove the nucleus prior to cracking. Decreasing the total ultrasound energy required to emulsify the nucleus presumably reduces injury to the corneal endothelium.

In our experience thus far, the procedure appears safe and we have had no capsular ruptures during chopping. Nonetheless, the procedure requires fine motor control, mastery of the spatial relationships in the anterior segment, and substantial practice. The most significant potential risk of this procedure is to inadvertently place the choppers in the sulcus outside the lens capsule, thereby rupturing zonules and disinserting the capsular bag during chopping. The 2 mm length of the chopper's distal end helps to ensure that the central posterior capsule will be untouched. Furthermore, we have consistently noted that the epinuclear shell is completely smooth and intact following nuclear chopping, underscoring the avoidance of the posterior capsule during this procedure.

Using this technique of chopping and minimal phaco power, we have documented a high degree of corneal clarity and excellent subjective visual results on the first postoperative day.

We also find nuclear cracking or a combination of cracking and chopping to be useful in fragmenting the nucleus. The techniques of

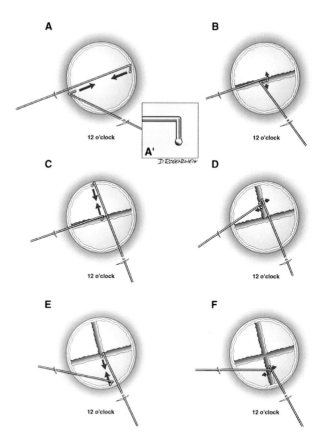

FIGURE 5–6. Kammenn Chopping Technique. **(A)** The choppers are inserted 90 degrees apart and positioned. **(B)** The two choppers are drawn together toward the visual axis. **(C)** The choppers are positioned on either of the heminucleus opposite to the cataract wound. **(D)** Choppers are carefully drawn together. **(E)** Choppers positioned on the proximal heminucleus. **(F)** Fractured into two quadrants.

nuclear bowling, sculpting or debulking are not recommended, however, as these techniques require the greatest amount of ultrasound and energy.

Aspiration of residual cortical material following nuclear evacuation should be done judiciously, trying to minimize the amount of irrigation fluid used. We use BSS Plus Sterile Irrigating Solution (Alcon) which contains specialized bicarbonate buffers, glutathione, and dextrose to help maintain endothelial cell integrity and viability. To each 500 ml bottle of BSS Plus we add 0.1 ml of 50 mg/ml vancomycin, 4 mg of gentamicin, 0.5 ml of 1:1000 epinephrine, and 0.8 ml of heparin (1000 units/ml) after passing each solution through a 0.22 um micropore filter.

BSS Plus is used sparingly at the end of the case to ensure a formed chamber while leaving the eye soft.

We do not advocate performing an astigmatic keratotomy at the time of cataract surgery in these patients.

■ Calculation of IOL Power in Triple Procedure

A triple procedure results in significant alterations of corneal curvature, anterior chamber depth, and axial length making IOL calculation less precise than for cataract surgery alone. Numerous techniques of IOL power calculation have been described for use in triple procedures, including the use of preoperative peripheral videokeratoscopic data of the recipient cornea.[5] We believe the most accurate method of IOL calculation is to use empirical nomograms personalized for each physician which relate average postoperative corneal curvature to the sizes of the donor button and the recipient bed.

Once personalized factors are taken into account, a variety of IOL power formulas may be used including SRK II (our formula of choice), SRK/T, Holladay 1, and Hoffer Q as noted in a study by CW Flowers et al.[6] When using SRK II, we subtract 0.50 to 1.00 D from the calculated lens power for high myopes and we add 0.50 to 1.00 D to the calculated lens power for high hyperopes. If the fellow eye has had prior cataract surgery with IOL, we use the difference between the actual and predicted refractions for the fellow eye in guiding our choice of lens power.

■ Postoperative Management

Patients should be informed that their vision may continue to improve 4 to 6 weeks or even longer after surgery due to sustained corneal edema. Patients need to be reassured during the postoperative period, as many of them will know of friends and family members without underlying corneal pathology who experienced more rapid visual recovery.

Ocular inflammation should be controlled quickly with judicious use of steroids. Initial therapy beginning on the first postoperative day consists of topical 1% prednisolone acetate QID. These steroid drops are generally tapered at weekly intervals to TID, BID, QD and then discontinued. Sodium chloride 5% drops QID during the day and 5% sodium chloride ointment at bedtime are often required for 3 to 4 weeks to treat initial postoperative corneal edema.

Intraocular pressure is maintained at low to normal levels postoperatively. Timolol maleate 0.5% BID and/or dorzolamide 2% TID are administered as needed to control IOP.

■ Tips and Pearls

1. Use adhesive viscoelastics liberally throughout the procedure to help protect the corneal endothelium.
2. When first learning the chopping technique, it may be helpful to groove and crack the nucleus at the outset and then use chopping to divide each heminucleus into quarters.
3. A widely dilated pupil and a large capsulorhexis (at least 6 mm in diameter) will facilitate anterior cortical removal and proper placement of the choppers.
4. Begin by aspirating as much anterior lens cortex as possible to prevent clouding of the view with cortical debris when chopping.
5. Keep chopping tips deep into the substance of the lens to achieve a complete chop. Perform the chopping motions in a smooth, slow, and controlled fashion to avoid rotating the nucleus within the capsular bag.
6. Once the nucleus is cleaved, use choppers to pull fragments in opposite directions to propagate the division along the entire lens thickness.
7. Additional I/A may be helpful after the first chop to restore a clear view.
8. Once the phaco tip is imbedded into a nuclear quadrant, maintain complete tip occlusion when using aspiration (foot position 2) to pull nuclear fragments centrally. Even a small amount of ultrasound during this maneuver will compromise the seal between the phaco tip and the nucleus, resulting in a loss of vacuum, regardless of machine parameters.
9. Concentrate on using the second instrument to mechanically divide the nucleus as much as possible to reduce the total ultrasound energy required. Endocapsular emulsification of quadrants with the phaco tip in the bevel down position may help to protect the corneal endothelium from dissipated ultrasound energy.
10. Begin with softer nuclei; denser lenses will require more practice and skill.

■ Acknowledgments

Special thanks to Eric D. Donnenfeld, M.D. for providing all the slit lamp photos for this chapter.

REFERENCES

1. Adamis AP, Filatov V, Tripathi BJ, Tripathi RC. Fuchs' endothelial dystrophy of the cornea. Surv Ophthalmol 1993;38:149–168.
2. Albert DM and Jakobiec FA. Principles and Practice of Ophthalmology. Philadelphia: W.B. Saunders; 1994; 51–54.
3. Pineros OE, Cohen EJ, Rapuano CJ, Laibson PR. Triple vs. nonsimultaneous procedures in Fuchs' dystrophy and cataract. Arch Ophthalmol 1996;114:525–528.
4. Malbran ES, Malbran E, Buonsanti J, Adrogue E. Closed-system phacoemulsification and posterior chamber implant combined with penetrating keratoplasty. Ophthalmic Surg 1993;24:403–406.
5. Serdaravic ON, Renard GJ, Pouliquen Y. Videokeratoscopy of recipient peripheral corneas in combined penetrating keratoplasty, cataract extraction, and lens implantation. Am J Ophthalmol 1996;122:29–37.
6. Flowers CW, McLeod SD, McDonnell PJ, et al. Evaluation of intraocular lens power calculation formulas in the triple procedure. J Cataract Refract Surg 1996;22: 116–122.

6

Intraocular Lens Power Calculation in Triple Procedures

OLIVIA N. SERDAREVIC

Advances in intraocular lens (IOL) power calculations, equipment for measuring preoperative parameters, and cataract surgical techniques enable surgeons to achieve spherical equivalent refractive results within ±0.50 D of emetropia in 90% of cases.[1] IOL power calculations have improved because of improved predictability of effective lens position (ELP), resulting from multiple-variable prediction formulas and more consistent capsular IOL implantation.[2] IOL power calculations in patients who have undergone corneal surgery, such as keratorefractive surgery, are known to be less predictable since the measured corneal powers are usually greater than the true refractive power of the cornea and IOL formulas often use keratometry as a predictor.[2] IOL power calculations in patients who are simultaneously undergoing penetrating keratoplasty, cataract extraction, and IOL implantation are even more prone to error since the central corneal power of the donor cornea is never measured preoperatively, and postoperative central corneal power is very dependent on individual surgical technique. Refractive results after triple procedures (Tables 6–1 and 6–2) cannot match those after cataract surgery alone, since accurate prediction of postoperative corneal curvature is necessary for accurate IOL calculation. Nonetheless, refinements in corneal transplantation techniques and instrumentation combined with an increased number of preoperative variables that can be measured and effectively used to calculate IOL power have improved refractive outcomes after triple procedures in recent years.[3–6]

Axial length was found to be the most important determining factor for accurate IOL calculation in triple procedures.[7,8] This variable is no longer the major source of error after procedures because of improvements in ultrasonic biometric measurement of axial length. The most important factor after axial length was shown by multiple regression analysis to be postoperative keratometry.[8]

Postoperative corneal power was not even considered in the 1970s when surgeons used a standard-power IOL.[9] Preoperative keratometry values of the operated or contralateral eye were used for IOL power calculations in the 1980s,[10] despite the lack of any correlation between preoperative and postoperative central corneal powers.[6,10,11] This lack of correlation is logical, since keratometry measures only the central portion of a recipient cornea which is removed at the time of penetrating keratoplasty.

TABLE 6–1. Range of Predictive Error After Triple Procedures

Study (Year)	Maximal Myopic Shift	Maximal Hyperopic Shift
Katz and Forster (1985)*	−6.88	+7.89
Musch and Meyer(1988)†	−7.00	+7.00
Geggel(1990)‡	−3.87	+1.75
Serdarevic(1996)	−2.54	+1.22

*Multiple surgeons; simultaneous penetrating keratoplasty, cataract extraction, and intraocular 1 lens implantation.
†Single surgeon; simultaneous penetrating keratoplasty, cataract extraction, and intraocular lens implantation.
‡Single surgeon; penetrating keratoplasty with or without cataract extraction followed at least nine months later by cataract extraction with intraocular lens implantation or secondary intraocular implantation with wound revision.
Modified from: Serdarevic ON, Renard GJ, Pouliquen Y. Videokeratoscopy of recipient peripheral corneas in combined penetrating keratoplasty, cataract extraction, and lens implantation. Am J Ophthalmol 1996;122:29–37.

Some surgeons suggested developing regression formulas for IOL power calculations to improve refractive results in triple procedures,[7,8,12] but others found no statistical difference in refractive outcomes between use of a surgeon-specific formula compared with use of a standard formula with a surgeon-specific average postoperative keratometry value.[11] Future studies using personalized A constants or S factors with third generation IOL power formulas and newer cataract and corneal surgical techniques may show a refractive advantage.

Since the 1980s, many studies demonstrated that the difficulty of predicting postoperative central corneal power was the main cause of an unintended refractive error after triple procedures.[7-23] Refractive results after triple procedures were documented to be superior when triple procedures were performed by a single surgeon using a standardized technique and calculating IOL power with the surgeon's average postoperative keratometry values than when performed by multiple surgeons using multiple techniques.[6,11,22] In the studies in which a single surgeon used average keratometry readings, 67 to 88% of patients attained a spherical equivalent refractive error within 2 D of the intended result, whereas only 26 to 49% of patients in studies with multiple surgeons and techniques achieved these results.

Very few studies to date have compared IOL power calculation formulas in triple procedures. Flowers and associates found no difference in predictability of postoperative refractive results in triple procedures when using several second- and third-generation formulas.[24] However, since the study was retrospective and included results of multiple surgeons using multiple techniques with postoperative spherical equivalent refractive errors ranging from −11.00 to +12.00 D, a study comparing the latest-generation formulas and clarifying their roles in refractive errors has yet to be performed. Theoretically, third-generation formulas that adjust ELP for varying axial length and corneal curvatures should give superior refractive results in triple procedures than second-generation formulas that adjust ELP only for varying axial lengths. The Sanders-Retzlaff-Kraff / T (SRK/T) multiple regression analysis formula without personalized A constants was used recently in a prospective clinical trial in which the postoperative refractive errors ranged from −2.54 to +1.22 D. Future multiple-variable prediction formulas should improve refractive outcomes even further.

It is only recently[6] that a study identified preoperative recipient corneal measurements that could be used reliably as an indicator of

TABLE 6–2. Spherical Equivalent Refractive Error Within ±2 D of Desired Result after Triple Procedures

Study (Year)	Eyes Within ±2 D (%)
Katz and Forster (1985)*	(26)
Binder (1985)	(49)
Binder (1986)	(56)
Musch and Meyer (1988)	(67)
Mattax and McCulley (1989)†	(63)
Mattax and McCulley (1989)‡	(82)
Binder (secondary intraocular lens) (1989)	(68)
Geggel (secondary intraocular lens) (1990)	(95)
Serdarevic (1996)	(88)

*Multiple surgeons.
†All patients; N + 16
‡Only patients for whom the surgeon's average postkeratoplasty keratometry values were used with the Sanders-Retzlaff-Kraff /T.
Modified from: Serdarevic ON, Renard GJ, Pouliquen Y. Videokeratoscopy of recipient peripheral corneas in combined penetrating keratoplasty, cataract extraction, and lens implantation. Am J Ophthalmol 1996;122:29–37.

postoperative outcomes, since, prior to that study, no investigation demonstrated a significant correlation between any preoperative measurement of recipient corneas and any postoperative measurement of grafted corneas.[7-23]

Serdarevic and associates first evaluated the influence of recipient peripheral corneas on refractive power of grafted donor corneas after triple procedures and demonstrated a significant correlation between preoperative dioptric power of peripheral recipient corneas and postoperative central power of grafted corneas.[6] Prior to that study, the only recipient corneal measurements that were used for IOL power calculations were keratometry values.

Serdarevic and collaborators used computerized videokeratoscopy to analyze the peripheral portion of recipient corneas.[6] In that study, an eye was arbitrarily classified as having a flat peripheral cornea when, at the circumference of the map, corneal powers were of less than 40.0 D in more than one clock hour (Fig. 6–1). An eye was classified as having a steep peripheral cornea when less than one clock hour of the circumference of the map or when no area of the map demonstrated dioptric powers of less than 40.0 D. Some eyes that were classified as having flat peripheral corneas had higher central dioptric powers that other eyes that were classified as having steep peripheral corneas. When videokeratoscopic analysis demonstrated a steep peripheral cornea, 46.00 D/46.00 D (the surgeon's average postoperative central corneal power) was used in the IOL power calculation formula. When videokeratoscopic analysis showed a flat cornea, 45.00 D/45.00 D (1 D flatter than the surgeon's postoperative central corneal power) was used to avoid postoperative hyperopic shifts and to decrease deviation from the desired refractive outcome.

Analysis of covariance demonstrated a strong correlation ($P = 0.0001$) between preoperative peripheral dioptric powers of the recipient cornea on the corneal maps and the postoperative central corneal power and no correlation between preoperative central corneal power and postoperative central corneal power. Since dioptric power measurements of the peripheral cornea obtained by videokeratoscopy could be used as indicators of postoperative central corneal power, these measurements could be used to effectively modify the average postoperative corneal power employed in IOL power calculations.

It should be emphasized that the videokeratoscopic data in that study was used as dioptric power measurements and not as corneal shape measurements, since software based on tangential analysis was not available at the

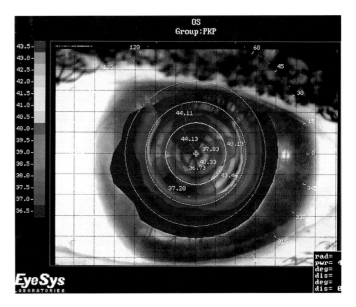

FIGURE 6–1. Corneal map of eye with flat peripheral cornea demonstrating peripheral dioptric powers under 37.00 D and a central corneal power of 42.41 D.

time of the study. Moreover, the peripheral dioptric power measurements obtained in the study were used as indicators rather than the true refractive powers since the available software did not take into consideration spherical aberration using Snell's law. Effective refractive powers of the peripheral cornea obtained by using current software such as the Holladay software (Corneal Analysis System, EyeSys Laboratories), which takes into consideration spherical aberration, would be approximately 2 D greater than dioptric powers of the same region used in the study of Serdarevic and associates. In other words, 42 D rather than 40 D might have been the value determining flat and steep peripheral corneas. A surgeon should determine the differentiating value for flat and steep peripheral corneas based on his or her own technique and average postoperative central corneal powers. Improvements in algorithms for videokeratoscopic measurement of peripheral corneal power, as well as improvements in nonvideokeratoscopic techniques for quantifying peripheral corneal shape, may improve prediction of postoperative corneal power even further.

To date, the influence of donor corneas on postoperative refractive outcome has not been adequately studied. Although Dave and McCulley[25] demonstrated that an automated portable keratometer can measure reproducibly central corneal powers of cadaveric donor corneas and suggested the feasibility of incorporating these measurements to predict postoperative refractive outcome, eye banks routinely do not measure corneal curvatures of donor corneas.

Improvements in prediction of postoperative central corneal power in triple procedures combined with improvements in cataract surgery, such as capsulorhexis that ensures more reproducible anteroposterior placement of the IOL, and with improvements in keratoplasty techniques, such as intraoperative suture adjustment that more reliably controls astigmatism[3-5] allow surgeons to achieve goals after triple procedures with as much accuracy as after staged procedures that may increase visual rehabilitation time and safety risks.[6,26,27]

■ Tips and Pearls

1. Use third-generation formulas for your IOL power calculations. The more preoperative variables you can measure, the more improved refractive outcomes you will obtain after triple procedures.
2. Remember that the difficulty of predicting postoperative central corneal power is the main cause of an unintended refractive error after triple procedures.
3. Use the Holladay software for the EyeSyS Corneal Analysis System to determine if the recipient cornea has a flat (<42 D in more than one clock hour) or steep periphery (when less than one clock hour of the circumference of the map or when no area of the map demonstrated dioptric powers <42 D).
4. When videokeratoscopic analysis demonstrated a steep peripheral cornea, 46.00/46.00 D is used in the IOL power calculation formula.
5. When a videokeratoscopic analysis shows a flat peripheral cornea, 45.00/45.00 D is then used for the IOL power calculation.
6. The surgeon should determine the differentiating value for flat and steep peripheral corneas based on his or her own technique and average postoperative central corneal powers.

REFERENCES

1. Brint SF. Refractive cataract surgery. Int Ophthalmol Clin 1994;34:1–11.
2. Holladay JT. Intraocular lens power calculations for cataract and refractive surgery. In: Serdarevic O. Refractive Surgery: Current Techniques and Management. New York: Igaku-Shoin Medical Publishers, Inc.; 1997.
3. Serdarevic ON. Refractive corneal transplantation: control of astigmatism and ametropia during penetrating keratoplasty. Int Opthalmol Chin 1994;34:13–33.
4. Serdarevic ON, Renard GJ, Pouliquen Y. Randomized clinical trial comparing astigmatism and visual rehabilitation after penetrating keratoplasty with and without intraoperative suture adjustment. Ophthalmology 1994;101:990–999.
5. Serdarevic ON, Renard GJ, Pouliquen Y. Randomized clinical trial of penetrating keratoplasty: before and after suture removal comparison of intraoperative

and postoperative suture adjustment. Ophthalmology 1995;102:1497–1503.
6. Serdarevic ON, Renard GJ, Pouliquen Y. Videokeratoscopy of recipient peripheral corneas in combined penetrating keratoplasty, cataract extraction, and lens implantation. Am J Ophthalmol 1996;122:29–37.
7. Binder PS. Intraocular lens powers used in the triple procedure: effect on visual acuity and refractive error. Ophthalmology 1985;92:1561–1566.
8. Crawford GJ, Stulting RD, Waring GO, Van Meter WS, Wilson LA. The triple procedure: analysis of outcome, refraction, and intraocular lens power calculation. Ophthalmology 1986;93:817–824.
9. Taylor DM. Keratoplasty and intraocular lenses. Ophthalmic Surg 1976;7:31–42.
10. Katz HR, Forster RK. Intraocular lens calculations in combined penetrating keratoplasty, cataract extraction and intraocular lens implantation. Ophthalmology 1985;92:1203–1207.
11. Musch DC, Meyer RF. Prospective evaluation of a regression determined formula for use in triple procedure surgery. Ophthalmology 1988;95:79–85.
12. Binder PS. The triple procedure: refractive results, 1985 update. Opthhalmology 1986;93:1482–1488.
13. Lee JR, Dohlman CH. Intraocular lens implantation in combination with keratoplasty. Ann Ophthalmol 1977;9:513–518.
14. Aquavella JV, Shaw EL, Rao GN. Intraocular lens implantation combined with penetrating keratoplasty. Ophthalmic Surg 1977; 8:113–116.
15. Buxton JN, Jaffe MS. Combined keratoplasty, cataract extraction and intraocular lens implantation. Am Intraocular Implant Soc J 1978; 4:110.
16. Taylor DM, Khaliq A, Maxwell R. Keratoplasty and intraocular lenses: current status. Ohtalmology 1979; 86:242–255.
17. Gould HL. Keratoplasty and intraocular lenses. Am Introcular Implant Soc J 1980; 6:42–44.
18. Bruner WE, Stark WJ, Maumenee AE. Combined keratoplasty, cataract extraction, and intraocular lens implantation: experience at the Wilmer Institute. Opththalmic Surg1981;12:657–660.
19. Lindstrom RL, Harris WS, Doughman DJ. Combined penetrating keratoplasty, extracapsular cataract extraction, and posterior chamber lens implantation. Am Intraocular Implant Soc J 1981;7:130–132.
20. Hunkeler JD, Hyde LL. The triple procedure: combined penetrating keratoplasty, cataract xtraction and lens implantation. Am Intraocular Implant Soc J 1983;9:20–24.
21. Pradera I, Ibrahim O, Waring GO. Refractive results of successful penetrating keratoplasty: intraocular lens implantation with selective suture removal. Refract Corneal Surg 1989;5:231–239.
22. Mattax JB, McCulley JP. The effect of standardized keratoplasty technique on IOL power calculation for the triple procedure. Acta Ophthalmol 1989;67 Suppl 192:24–29.
23. Claoue C, Ficker L, Kirkness C, Steele A. Refractive results after corneal triple procedures (PK+ECCE+IOL). Eye 1993;7:446–451.
24. Flowers CW, McLeod SD, McDonnell PJ, Irvine JA, Smith RE. Evaluation of intraocular lens power calculation formulae in the triple procedure. ARVO abstracts. Invest Ophthalmol Vis Sci 1994;35(4,suppl):1874.
25. Dave AS, McCulley JP. Demonstration of feasibility of application of a portable keratometer to cadaveric donor corneas. Cornea 1994;13:379–382.
26. Binder PS. Intraocular lens implantation after penetrating keratoplasty. Refract Corneal Surg 1989;5: 224–230.
27. Geggel HS. Intraocular lens implantation after penetrating keratoplasty: improved unaided visual acuity, astigmatism, and safety in patients with combined corneal disease and cataract. Ophthalmology 1990; 97:1460–1467.

7

Management of the Small Pupil in Phacoemulsification

VIRGILIO CENTURIÓN, I. HOWARD FINE, AND LUIS W. LU

Phacoemulsification in Difficult and Challenging Cases
Edited by Luis W. Lu and I. Howard Fine.
Thieme Medical Publishers, Inc.,
New York, ©1999.

Good mydriasis is one of the necessary conditions to perform safe cataract surgery. However, there are situations when pupils do not dilate or dilate poorly.

Recently dramatic advancements have happened, and a number of techniques were developed to provide good mydriasis for surgery.

Besides surgery facilitation, the main objective of these techniques is to allow the normal functioning of the pupil without causing functional or esthetic changes that can compromise the final results.

The small pupil was considered a contraindication for the beginning phaco surgeon. With the development of new techniques and equipment, the small pupil phacoemulsification is now considered as a "more delicate" surgery with highly predictable results.

Gimbel and Col[1] reported an incidence of 1.6% of small pupil in a group of 1880 consecutive phacoemulsification surgeries.

■ Preoperative Considerations

Assessment of the pupil, dynamically and statically, during preoperative examination is very important. A simple, dynamic evaluation includes observation of the pupil under different levels of light intensity: half-shadow, darkness, and direct light. This procedure has extreme practical value.

When talking about "static" evaluation we are referring to an examination after the use of mydriatic drops for a diagnostic purpose: phenylephrine 10%—1 drop, and tropicamide 1%—1 drop and after 20 to 30 minutes the size of the pupil is evaluated. Both static and dynamic observations are performed under the slit lamp.

After assessment, the conclusions could be a pupil with optimal, good, regular, or poor reaction to the mydriatics agents or a pupil with no reaction to a mydriatic drug remaining small, unaltered. But what is a small pupil? A small pupil is the one with a diameter under 4 mm that can be a cause of complication during phacoemulsification. However, this diameter is not a contraindication for the experienced surgeon.

Considering these observations, we suggest a classification of small pupils as follows: Functional, or hyporeactive, or lazy pupil; and Anatomical, or fixed pupil.

The *hyporeactive* pupil dilates under pharmacological mydriasis but in an unsatisfactory way. They are more frequent among high hyperopic eyes, constantly medicated patients or elderly patients with those individual characteristics.

The *fixed* pupil does not react during dynamic examination, and no reaction to mydriatic drugs has many causes, the most common being senile, inflammatory (after uveitis), traumatic, miosis following neurological diseases, and iatrogenic miosis (chronic usage of miotic drug for the treatment of glaucoma). Regardless of the cause, it is *usual* to attribute the presence of a structural change in these cases of small and fixed pupil of long duration. Among these structural changes are arteriosclerosis, hyalinization of the iris stroma, and dilator muscle atrophy.

The preoperative classification facilitates the treatment strategy for the small pupil during phacoemulsification (Table 7–1). According to the type of small pupil (previously determined), the most adequate technique is used for obtaining a good mydriasis during surgery.

In a retrospective study of 1802 consecutive phacoemulsification procedures, the author found a 1.77% (32 eyes) incidence of small pupil. The most common surgical complication was posterior capsular rupture with an incidence of 0.22%.

TABLE 7–1. Classification of Small Pupil Type and Most Appropriate Technique.

Pupil	Technique

Functional or Hyporeactive	Pharmacologic
	Viscoelastc agent
	Mechanical: Hooks
	    Mackool
	    De Juan
	    Iris Ring
	    Bheeler Pupil Dilator
	    Keuch Pupil Dilator

Anatomical or Fixed	Mechanical
	    Hooks
	    Stretch Pupiloplasty
	    Iris Ring
	    Bheeler pupil dilator
	Incisional
	    Sphincterotomy
	    Iridotomy
	      Superior
	      Inferior
	    Iridectomy

■ Surgical Techniques

The Hyporeactive Pupil

The "lazy pupil" is usually found in high hyperopic eyes (with axial length of less than 22.0 mm) or in patients with senile miotic pupil. In these cases, pharmacologic dilation yields a pupil of approximately 4 mm or less, increasing the risk of complications during phacoemulsification. The capsulorhexis will be very small, nucleus manipulation risky, and the intraocular lens (IOL) implantation will be difficult. We recommend the following techniques and sequence of their application.

Pharmacologic Treatment

If it is known after the preoperative examination that the pupil will be poorly dilated, we ask the nursing staff to use the "maximum dosage cocktail of mydriatics", that is the administration of Phenylephrine 10%, Tropicamide 1% (Mydriacyl[R]), and Ketorolac Tromethamine 0.5% (Acular[R]) or Flurbiprofen 0.03% (Ocufen[R]) three times (nine drops total) starting one hour prior to surgery, and maintenance of the patient in a dimly lit room. The use of cyclopentolate (Cyclogyl[R]) is not recommended because of its possible psychogenic side effects. Once at surgery if the obtained mydriasis is less than 4 mm, 0.5 ml of unpreserved adrenaline 1:1000 diluted in 10 ml of BSS is introduced through the paracentesis incision. After the main incision is completed, and if the dilation obtained is not acceptable, we proceed to the second method, the use of *"heavy viscoelastic agent,"* a highly viscous, elastic, and pseudoplastic agent. A 4 mm pupil does not constitute a contraindication for the experienced surgeon to perform endocapsular phacoemulsification. The small capsulorhexis could be enlarged after the IOL implantation to prevent its retraction (phimosis) postoperatively. In these cases it is very important the use of the bimanual technique with the iris manipulator or the nucleus rotator for stretching the iris during phacoemulsification.[2]

If after the use of the viscoelastic agent, a 5 to 6 mm stable pupil is obtained, the bimanual and

CHAPTER 7 ■ Management of the Small Pupil

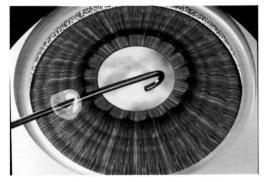

FIGURE 7–1. Placement of an iris hook through a paracentesis.

Mechanical Treatment with IrisHooks[4,5,7,8]

These hooks, in soft and flexible nylon (Figs. 7–1 to 7–5), are introduced after four symmetrical incisions placed at 10, 2, 5, and 7 o'clock positions. After the scleral or corneal tunnels are developed and the viscoelastic material injected, these secondary incisions should be performed with the symmetrical introduction of the hooks (i.e., first 2 o'clock; second 7 o'clock, third 5 o'clock, and 10 o'clock). We "hook" the pupillary margin, and then its retraction is carefully forced towards the iris periphery, where it will be fixated with the help of the hook's adjusting silicone sleeve. After good positioning of the hooks and assessment of the mydriasis are obtained, the surgery is performed in its usual sequence. Immediately after IOL implantation, the hooks are carefully removed (very flexible, nontraumatic) and self-sealing closure of the incisions is evaluated.

endocapsular phacoemulsification technique will be quite safe. Failure of the above mentioned methods led us to the use of mechanical forms of treatment, as the De Juan iris hooks,[4,5] or the Beehler pupil dilator[6] (Table 7–2, p. 59).

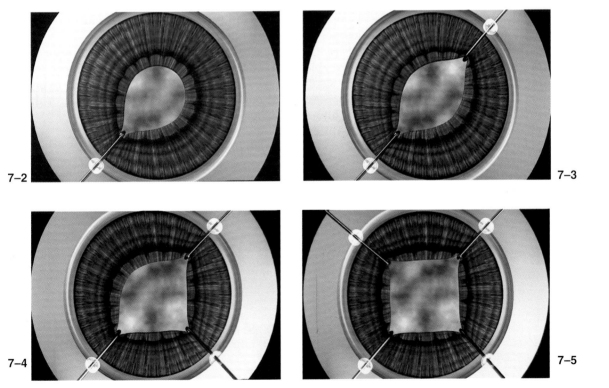

FIGURES 7–2 to 7–5 (surgeon's view). Appearance of the pupil as one, two, three, and four hooks have been placed and the retaining silicone sleeve is tightened to the site of the paracentesis.

Beehler Pupil Dilator[6] (Moria#19009)

At present, we find this instrument to be uniformly applicable in the presence of small pupils. Inserted through the cataract incision, the proximal iris is engaged with a mounted hook on the undersurface of the instrument and retracted while the dilator is opened to stretch the pupil at four points on 360 degrees. It usually stretches the pupil 5.0 to 7.0 mm while creating tiny microsphincterotomies circumferentially around the pupil (Fig. 7-6 to 7-8). The pupil diameter can then be mechanically reduced at the end of the procedure with a Lester hook supplemented with an intraocular miotic agent. Pupils enlarged in this manner maintain a good cosmetic appearance and an ability to react to light but may require miotic drops for some time after cataract surgery to avoid synechias to the capsulorhexis margin.

The Keuch Pupil Dilator (Katena K3-4950)

Can be used in a similar manner. This instrument is designed to enlarge a small pupil in preparation for cataract surgery. It features a narrow cannulated tip with one fixed iris retractor for pulling the iris and one moveable central stem for pushing the iris. It is small enough to be used through a sideport incision as well as the primary cataract incision, allowing the surgeon to dilate the iris in two different quadrants with one instrument.

These options have facilitated the performance of cataract surgery especially in eyes without anatomical problems, that is, in which

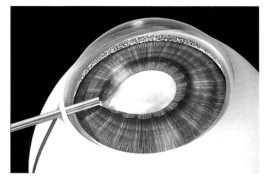

FIGURE 7-7. Engaging the subincisional pupil with the hook on the bottom of the Beehler pupil dilator.

proper mydriasis is not obtained because of functional causes.

The Fixed Pupil

In presence of hyporeactive pupils, it is often necessary to use mechanical methods to obtain good mydriasis. Using the proper techniques will lead to good postoperative aesthetics and pupillary function.

The most acceptable methods are mechanical and among the mechanical pupil expanders we prefer the Stretch Pupiloplasty with the "pull and push" technique as well as the use of the Beehler pupil dilator.

Stretch Pupiloplasty [2,3]

Two secondary paracentesis are made 90° away from the main incision. With the anterior chamber filled with viscoelastic material, the

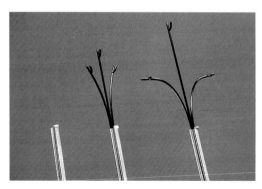

FIGURE 7-6. Beehler pupil dilator.

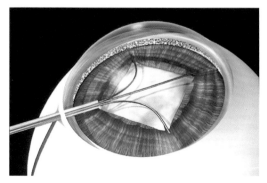

FIGURE 7-8. Full extension of the retractor arms of the Beehler pupil dilator.

TABLE 7–2. Management of the Hyporeactive Pupil

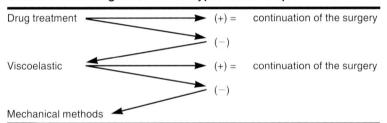

dilators or two Graether collar buttons[16] are introduced through the two secondary incisions (9 and 3 o'clock in the case of the 12 o'clock location for the cataract incision), and after fixation at the pupillary margin (Fig. 7–9), traction is made away from the incisions in the direction of the iris periphery (Figs. 7–10, and 7–11). That traction must be done with gentle, firm, and continuous movements to a point close to the irido-corneal angle.

Then, one of the retractors is removed (the 3 o'clock on the right eye, and the 9 o'clock on the left eye) and introduced through the main incision (Fig. 7–12). The 12 o'clock pupillary margin is captured with one retractor, and the 6 o'clock is approached with the other to perform a similar maneuver in the 6–12 o'clock direction as previously described (Fig. 7–12).

Immediately after removing the retractors, the anterior chamber is filled with viscoelastic material, the pupil diameter is verified and the surgery is then continued in a safe and comfortable manner. Occasionally slight

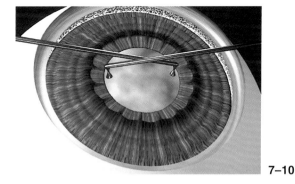

7–10

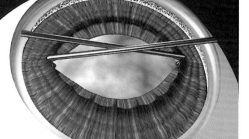

7–11

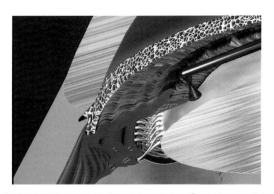

FIGURE 7–9. Relationship of the Graether collar button to the pupillary margin.

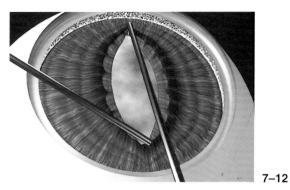

7–12

FIGURES 7–10 to 7–12. Engagement and stretching of the pupil in perpendicular meridians.

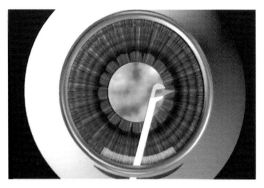

FIGURE 7–13. Initial partial sphincterotomy by Rapazzo scissors.

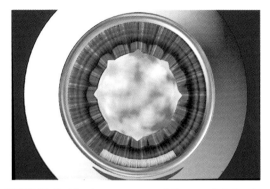

FIGURE 7–15. Appearance of the pupil following stretching of each of the sphincterotomy sites.

bleeding can be observed at the stretching site.

We prefer these techniques because they do not affect the pupillary function postoperatively and for its simplicity, reusable material, and low cost.

In the absence of proper armamentarium for mechanical methods, the most adequate incisional technique would be the *Multiple Sphincterotomies* (Pupilloplasty) (Figs. 7–13 to 7–15).

Pupilloplasty

The anterior chamber must be filled with viscoelastic material. Posterior synechias should be swept with a cyclodyalisis spatula. The Rapazzo scissors are introduced through the main cataract incision and we begin the systematic snipping of the pupillary edge, with incisions of 0.5 to 0.75 mm at regular intervals, being careful to not transect the full width of the sphincter muscle.

Following eight sphincterotomies, each of the sphincterotomied sites is stretched to the root of the iris with a Graether collar button or a Lester hook. This ruptures the fibrotic elements and stretches the muscular portion of the iris. Postoperatively, the cosmetic and physiologic function of the pupil is considered excellent.

We will now present illustrations of other techniques recommended in the literature by different authors.

The Mackool Technique

Mackool has designed self-retaining titanium hooks that can be placed through paracentesis so that the pupil can be positioned and held in a dilated state. The titanium hooks are placed and the pupil is then manipulated with a sec-

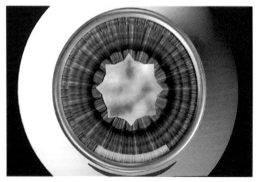

FIGURE 7–14. Appearance of the pupil following eight small sphincterotomies.

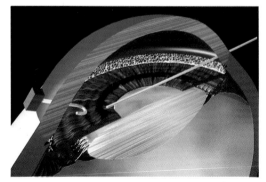

FIGURE 7–16. Mackool self-retaining hooks and iris pusher.

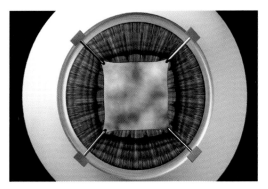

FIGURE 7–17. Appearance of the pupil with Mackool hooks in position.

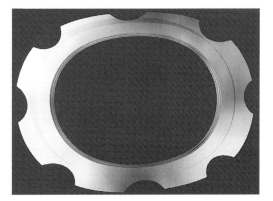

FIGURE 7–19. Almost completely hydrated iris protector ring.

ond instrument so that it can be stretched and placed into the hook from a paracentesis or through the main incision (Figs. 7–16 and 7–17).[6]

The Iris Protector Ring
Siepser designed a hydrogel ring which in its dehydrated form collapses to the configuration of a compressed oval.[5] It can be placed in its dehydrated form through a 3 mm incision and inserted into the pupil. The device expands with hydration. Because it has flanges on the edges of the inner surface, it captures the pupil and can be manipulated to expand it as the device expands. At the completion of the procedure, it can be removed with a hook through the same small incision (Figs. 7–18 to 7–21).[5]

The Partial Sphincterectomy
A partial sphincterectomy can be performed by grasping the superior sphincter and pulling it out of the incision. A segment of the sphincter can then be excised, after which the iris is repositioned. This results in a permanently large pupil that may be somewhat oval in shape, but frequently achieves adequate dilation for completion of the surgery (Figs. 7–22 and 7–23).[5]

Inferior Sphincterectomy
Masket has described a technique for using a pre-placed suture in the inferior distal portion of the iris, drawing a loop of the central segment of the suture out of the incision and then performing a sphincterectomy inferiorly. After implantation of the intraocular lens, the ends of the sutures are drawn out of the inferior or distal limbal self-sealing paracentesis and tied. This can dramatically increase exposure to the area in which most of the phacoemulsification takes place, i.e., the distant

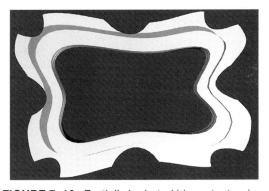

FIGURE 7–18. Partially hydrated iris protector ring.

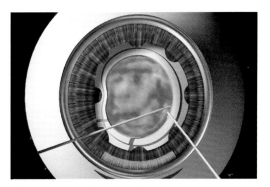

FIGURE 7–20. Manipulating the iris protector ring so that the flanges engage the pupil.

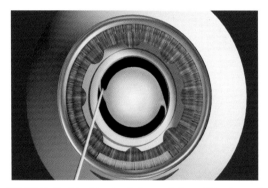

FIGURE 7–21. Manipulation of the IOL through the iris protector ring.

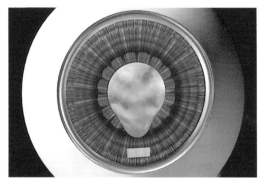

FIGURE 7–23. Enlargement of the pupil following partial sphincterotomy.

quadrant of the pupil, and can restore an acceptable cosmetic appearance postoperatively (Figs. 7–24 to 7–27).[11]

Superior Sector Iridectomy

A superior sector iridectomy is frequently used for pupillary enlargement. This technique subjects patients to glare and undesirable retinal images postoperatively because of the permanently dilated pupil and the potential for edge effects from the lens and haptics uncovered by the iridectomy. A modification of the iridectomy, which tends to give adequate dilation for surgery and is less of a problem postoperatively, is the superior mid-iris iridectomy followed by sphincterotomy. This allows the pillars of the iris to come together more closely following completion of the surgery than does a sector iridectomy. Many surgeons use a suture to close the sphincterectomy at the completion of the surgery hoping to avoid potential sources of glare and trying to achieve a more cosmetically acceptable appearance postoperatively (Figs. 7–28 to 7–33).[5]

These sutures may be pre-placed through a clear cornea. The posterior loop is drawn out of the peripheral iridectomy with a hook prior to sphincterotomy. Alternatively, the suture may be placed through clear cornea at the end of the procedure. The ends are drawn out of the cataract incision and tied.

■ Postoperative Considerations

The manipulation of a small pupil during cataract surgery can present some problems. Among the most common are an increase in inflammation of the anterior segment observed during the immediate postoperative period, light bleeding without clinical translation, light ocular hypertension secondary to

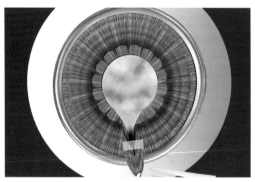

FIGURE 7–22. Excising a portion of the sub-incisional sphincter.

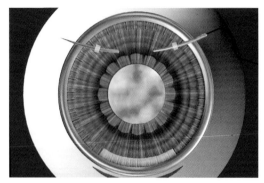

FIGURE 7–24. Pre-placement through clear cornea of an iris suture distally.

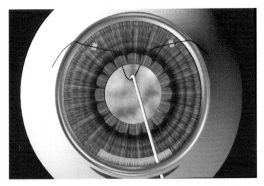

FIGURE 7–25. Retrieval of central loop of the suture from under the iris and through the incision.

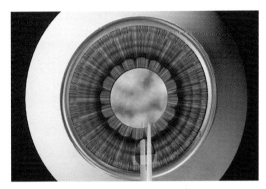

FIGURE 7–29. Transecting the residual iris to create a sector iridectomy.

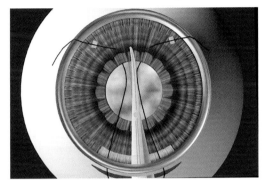

FIGURE 7–26. Inferior sphincterectomy.

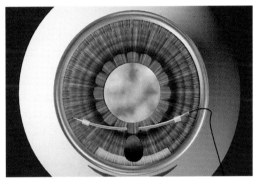

FIGURE 7–30. Needle passed through clear cornea, iris, and back out through clear cornea on the other side.

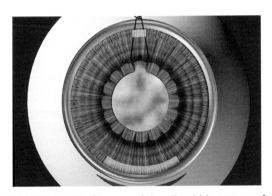

FIGURE 7–27. Closure of the distal iris suture after lens implantation.

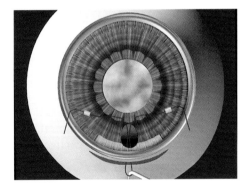

FIGURE 7–31. Central loop pulled through the peripheral iridotomy and out of the incision.

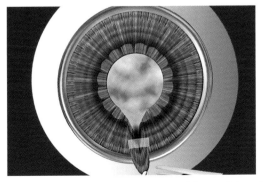

FIGURE 7–28. Excising a portion of the peripheral iris for peripheral iridotomy.

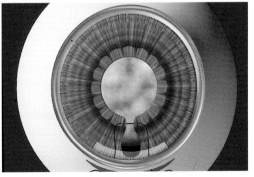

FIGURE 7–32. Both ends of the suture retrieved through the cataract incision after removing the needles and transecting the pupil through the iridectomy.

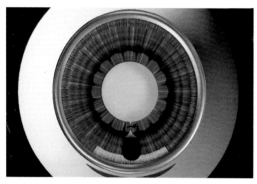

FIGURE 7–33. Tying the iris suture after lens implantation.

the inflammatory reaction, temporary or permanent mydriasis, aesthetical changes, and a decrease in visual acuity because of glare.[12]

Finally, the use of the better viscoelastic agents, good instruments, diversity of techniques and experience, and popularization of phacoemulsification techniques among ophthalmologists have made possible that the results obtained in small pupil cataract surgery are similar to the those obtained in normal sized pupils.

■ Tips and Pearls

1. Determine the size of the pupil preoperatively. Apply a drop of phenylephrine 10% and tropicamide 1% and make note of the pupillary dilation obtained.
2. Classify the pupil as hyporeactive or fixed and be prepared for the most appropriate dilating technique.
3. Apply a full pharmacologic schedule of dilation starting one hour prior to the surgery. Administer Phenylephrine 10%, Tropicamide 1%, and Ketorolac 0.5% three times (nine drops total).
4. Consider the addition of intracameral unpreserved Adrenaline 1:1000 diluted in 10 cc of BSS, as the first step in the management of a small pupil.
5. Utilize a highly viscous, elastic, and pseudoplastic viscoelastic material as a second step.
6. The third step will be mechanical pupillary dilation. At the present time our preference is the use of the Beehler pupil dilator, the De Juan iris hooks, and the bimanual pupillary stretching technique.

■ Conclusion

We present the most commonly used techniques for handling the small pupil during phacoemulsification as well as the most used or preferred by the authors at present. Surgeon experience, common sense, and the least traumatizing technique with the least intraocular manipulation will bring the most benefits to the patient.

REFERENCES

1. Gimbel HV. Nucleofractis phacoemulsification through a small pupil. Can J Ophthalmol 1992;27:115–119.
2. Miller KM, Keener GT. Stretch pupilloplasty for small pupil phacoemulsification (letter). Am J Ophthalmol 1994;3:107–108.
3. Dinsmore SC. Modified stretch technique for small pupil phacoemulsification with topical anesthesia. J Cataract Surg 1996;22:27–30.
4. De Juan E, Hickingbotham D. Flexible iris retractor (letter). Am J Ophthalmol 1991;111:776–777.
5. Fine IH. Phacoemulsification in the presence of a small pupil. In: Steinert RF (ed). Cataract Surgery: Technique, Complications and Management. Philadelphia: W.B. Saunders; 1995;199–208.
6. Fine IH, Hoffman RS. Phacoemulsification in the presence of pseudoexfoliation: challenges and options. J Cataract Refract Surg 1997;23:160–165.
7. Mackool RJ. Small pupil enlargement during cataract extraction: a new method. J Cataract Refract Surg 1992;18:523–526.
8. Nichamin LD. Enlarging the pupil for cataract extraction using flexible nylon iris retractors. J Cataract Refract Surg 1993;19:793–796.
9. Fine IH. Pupilloplasty. In: Koch PS, Davison JA (eds). Textbook of Advanced Phacoemulsification Techniques, Thorofare, NJ: Slack;1990;91–97.
10. Fine IH. Pupilloplasty technique to improve cosmesis and preserve function after cataract surgery. In: Nordan LT, Maxwell WA, Davison JA (eds). The Surgical Rehabilitation of Vision. NY: Gower Medical Publishing; 1992;14.1–14.4.
11. Masket S. Preplaced inferior iris suture method for small pupil phacoemulsification. J Cataract Refract Surg 1992;18:518–522.
12. Masket S. Relationship between postoperative pupil size and disability glare. J Cataract Refract Surg 1992;18:506–507.

8

Phacoemulsification in Patients with Uveitis

JORGE L. ALÍO Y SANZ AND ENRIQUE CHIPONT

Patients with uveitis have cataracts more often and at an earlier age than the general population. Intraocular inflammatory phenomena, as well as the drugs used to control them are considered as main etiological agents. Cataract surgery in the patient with uveitis is one of the challenges with greatest number of unknown factors faced by the ophthalmologist. The uncertainty of the postoperative process, the existence of an underlying systemic pathology, the poor tolerance of intraocular lenses (IOLs) observed in some cases, and the many technical difficulties make the handling of these patients very difficult before, during, and after the cataract operation.

In general, the visual prognosis of the patient with uveitis will depend on the presence of pre- and postsurgical inflammation, on the quality and efficiency of the surgical procedure, and on the treatment of complications, that is, secondary glaucoma.

■ Specific Considerations Related to the Patient with Uveitis.

Cataract surgery in the patient with uveitis presents a number of challenges in the presurgical, intraoperative, and postsurgical stages.[1] The surgeon should remember the following considerations when dealing with patients with uveitis:

1. Good control of the underlying systemic disorder is required. In many cases, the presence of a base inflammatory pathology with long standing and unpredictable evolution will condition the existence of recurrent inflammation. Its medical control may even require a multidisciplinary approach for this purpose. Our personal approach will be explained further in this chapter.

2. Control of the ocular inflammation is needed prior to the surgical procedure. This preoperative control may require the use of topical or systemic steroids or immunosuppressive drugs. The treatment should be aimed at achieving a reduction in cellularity in the anterior chamber, as well as little or no vitreous activity. The inflammatory activity should be assessed only by the presence of cells in the anterior chamber and not just by the amount of flare present.

3. Cataract surgery is sometimes complicated by the presence of iris atrophy, sclerosis of the pupillary sphincter, cyclitic membranes, posterior synechiae, anterior capsular sclerosis, and possible hemorrhage from the iris and

angle neovascularization (Figs. 8–1 and 8–2). The surgery is certainly more difficult because the frequent presence of miosis refractory to pharmacological dilation, anterior and posterior synechia, and glaucoma. A precise and delicate surgery is mandatory. Keep in mind that surgery can exacerbate the underlying inflammatory process by the release of lens material and by the surgical trauma itself. It is then very important that the surgery should be performed in an "undisturbed" eye with an inflammatory reaction that has been controlled for at least three months prior to surgery.

4. The IOL selection is another challenge for the surgeon. Remember to choose the proper intraocular lens when applicable. The design, overall diameter, and configuration are also considerations and further details will be given in this chapter. The IOL must be placed in the bag when possible. Avoid IOL implantation in those patients considered not to be good candidates.[2,3]

5. The firm control of the postoperative inflammation is imperative. The necessary use of topical and in most cases, periocular and systemic steroids, can give rise to problems as steroid-dependent ocular hypertension and even problems related to the progressive and full withdrawal of them. The use of nonsteroidal antiinflammatory drugs is a step forward in the postoperative control of inflammation.

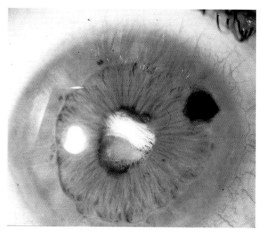

FIGURE 8–2. Cataract in a case of HLA B27 positive anterior uveitis. An anterior cyclitic membrane is frequent and usually associated to 360 degrees posterior synechia.

The postsurgical inflammatory reaction can produce a series of complications such as an increase in intraocular pressure, corneal edema, endothelial damage, secondary cataracts and postoperative macular edema, among others. The mechanical stimulation of the iris has been known to induce the release of prostaglandins E2 and F2a. Prostaglandins have been proven to play a role in ocular inflammatory reactions, particularly in those in which mechanical iris scraping has been performed.

The residues from polishing the intraocular lens during manufacturing were once another related cause of ocular inflammation, but is no longer the case because the high quality of modern IOL manufacturing.

Another factor that has been linked to postoperative tissue destruction is the activation of complement by the classic or alternative route. The activation of the alternative course has been known to start by the presence of intraocular lenses in contact with metabolically active tissues. Some polymers, especially prolene, cause activation of complement although some studies did not show a significant difference on activation of complement when comparing prolene with polymethylmethacrylate.[4] There are materials such as hydrogel which did not cause any significant activation of this factor.

In general, we would say that posterior chamber lenses designed for and placed in

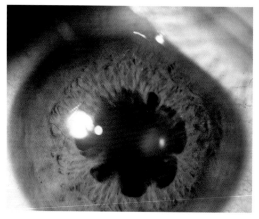

FIGURE 8–1. Nuclear and posterior subcapsular cataract in a case of idiopathic recurrent uveitis.

the capsular bag could reduce the possibility of mechanical irritation as compared with lenses designed for other locations.[5]

The introduction of phacoemulsification, viscoelastic materials, highly sophisticated instruments, and new IOL materials has reduced the number of complications in these patients.

■ Patient Preparation

Good pupillary dilation must be achieved when possible to avoid manipulation of the iris during surgery. However, surgical dilation may be required. Pupiloplasty with the Argon laser is not advisable. The De Juan disposable iris hooks work very well for very small pupils.

Angle neovascularization may be treated by argon laser focal photocoagulation at the area of the surgical incision. It is performed by using a 100 μ spot size, 0.2 sec of exposure, and enough energy to blanch the vessels in three different places along its course. Nevertheless, the cause of the neovascularization should be found and appropriate treatment given when applicable.

Proper control of the intraocular pressure is recommended 2 to 3 weeks prior to surgery. The use of cholinergic drugs should be avoided in these patients as they alter the hemato-aqueous barrier and tend to increase synechiae formation.

Control is generally obtained by using beta blockers and topical or occasionally systemic carbonic anhydrase inhibitors.

Preoperative hypotony in patients with uveitis can also be found and is frequently due to the formation of cyclitic membranes, ciliary body dialysis, and severe inflammation causing severe decrease in aqueous production. The destruction of the ciliary body itself is rarely found.

■ Preoperative Control of Inflammation

The use of topical and/or periocular steroids can be sufficient for handling both pre- and postoperative inflammation in a large number of patients. Although systemic steroid administration is controversial, one must recommend it to patients who have required systemic or periocular administration of steroids in a previous inflammatory stage. The administration of 60 to 80 mg/day of Prednisone must be considered, starting 2 weeks prior to the scheduled surgery. In general, the use of corticoids in children should not go beyond 3 months due to their possible side effects on growth.

If steroids alone are insufficient, immunosuppressive agents should be added.[6] These drugs have to be administered for at least 2 weeks prior to surgery because of their latency period. Among these drugs Methrotexate, Azathioprin, and Cyclosporin A are available.[7]

The following schedule is recommended:

1. Preparation should include full control of the underlying inflammatory process for at least 3 months prior to the scheduled surgery.
2. Prednisolone 1% should be added eight times a day starting 1 week before surgery.
3. One mg/kg/day of oral prednisone should be administered starting 1 week prior to the surgery, depending on the amount of inflammation.
4. Periocular steroid injection of Triamcinolone can help in handling severe inflammatory complications not controlled by topical or systemic medications.
5. Topical (Diclofenac 0.1%, Fulbiprofen 0.03%, Surprofen 1%) and systemic use of nonsteroidal antiinflammatory drugs (NSAIDS) is considered in cases of cystoid macular edema.[8]

■ Surgical Technique

If the uveitis has remained inactive, an anterior approach is undertaken, which is performed in the majority of cases. We prefer phacoemulsification for the cataract removal in these patients. Intracapsular surgery is reserved for the situations in which an important lens-induced component was present in a prior contralateral surgery.

If the inflammatory reaction persists or a chronic macular edema is present, a combined procedure should be performed—phacoemulsification and vitrectomy. Some authors have proposed performing this combined procedure from an anterior approach because the frequent presence of total vitreous detachment in these patients.[9] Most surgeons, opt for conventional pars plana vitrectomy techniques.[10,11]

Phacoemulsification

Phacoemulsification is our procedure of choice. It requires a small incision, causes minimal trauma, and minimizes postoperative inflammation. Young patients and patients on high doses of steroids benefit with this technique. General anesthesia is not necessary but is frequently requested by young patients. Local anesthesia by retrobulbar or peribulbar block are preferred. Topical anesthesia is not contraindicated but we prefer not to use it in these cases. Clear corneal incision is our preferred approach if no lens or a foldable lens is implanted, and if the implantation of a rigid PMMA lens is planned, a limbal approach with a short scleral tunnel is performed.

Viscoelastic materials are routinely used to release adhesions. The combination of hyaluronic acid and condroitin sulphate (Viscoat[R]) is preferred, but high viscosity materials (Healon GV[R], Amvisc plus[R]) can be used as well. Many patients with uveitis have sclerosis of the dilator muscle or severe posterior synechiae, and in these cases synechiolysis is performed with an iris spatula. If further mydriasis is desired, the flexible iris retractors are utilized. Continuous curvilinear capsulotomy (Capsulorhexis) is always attempted. If unsuccessful a can opener capsulotomy is done, but phacoemulsification is performed with caution.

Phaco chop techniques are used for removing a hard nucleus. In young patients with a soft nucleus, phacoaspiration may be all that is needed.

Intensive cortical clean up is mandatory to eliminate one of the sources of postoperative inflammatory reaction and the posterior surface of the anterior capsule must be vacuumed. Suturing the incision is advocated.[12]

There are some particular situations in which a prophylactic peripheral iridectomy may be recommended, as in cases of uveitis with high tendency for synechia formation, and possibly in all those who are to receive and intraocular lens, although the later is still a surgeon's decision. Patients in whom a vitrectomy have been performed with removal of the posterior capsule do not require an iridectomy.

In cases where there is an extensive membrane formation in the anterior vitreous, vitrectomy after posterior central capsulorhexis must be considered. If the vitreous cavity shows extensive fibrosis and exudate formation, transcleral pars plana vitrectomy may be indicated.

Combined Cataract-Vitrectomy Techniques

Pars plana vitrectomy combined with lensectomy can be the procedure of choice in cases of uveitis with vitreitis refractory to medical treatment. This technique can be useful in patients with chronic juvenile arthritis or pars planitis. Technically speaking, if the lensectomy is performed through pars plana vitrectomy, corneal distortion is avoided. However, some disadvantages are associated with this technique including the need for sulcus fixation of a posterior chamber IOL, the large discission needed in the residual anterior capsule, and the potential difficulties of aspirating residual cortical debris from the posterior surface of the anterior capsule. In addition, removal of a dense nuclear sclerotic cataract may be difficult to perform.

In our hands, the combined phacoemulsification and pars plana vitrectomy technique has many advantages over other techniques.[13,14]

IOL implantation after completion of the vitrectomy, if required, allows fast visual rehabilitation and functional unaided vision in patients who are considered poor candidates for aphakic contact lens wear.

If a limbal approach to the cataract and posterior pars plana vitrectomy is intended, the scleral incisions for the vitrectomy should be made first. The fixed infusion method and upper sclerotomies occluded with scleral plugs are utilized. A capsulotomy or posterior capsulorhexis must be performed upon completion of the vitrectomy because the high opacification rate and because it allows a free connection between the anterior and posterior segments of the eye, facilitating the access of anti-inflammatory drugs in the postoperative period.

Macular edema, retinal detachment, and glaucoma have been described as possible complications.[15,16]

Intraocular Lenses

Until recently, the existence of chronic uveitis has been regarded by most surgeons as a relative contraindication to IOL implantation.[17] For these reasons, sulcus or anterior chamber implantation has always been contraindicated and capsular bag placement has been controversial. On the other hand, several researchers have suggested that inserting a posterior chamber lens into the capsular bag poses no additional threat to ocular morbidity in selected uveitic eyes, provided proper perioperative treatment for inflammation is given.[18–20]

The use of anterior chamber IOLs should not be recommended in any type of uveitis. Some authors advocate the use of a single piece PMMA lenses in an attempt to prevent the activation of the complement which arises with polypropylene haptics.[21] Surface-modified IOLs such as the heparin coated models have also been introduced. The heparin surface-modified IOL is created by inducing electrostatic adsorption of heparin onto the surface of a PMMA IOL. Heparin coated IOLs are recommended for patients with uveitis as they decrease the number and severity of deposits on the surface of the IOL and although the IOL will not prevent or inhibit the development of fibrinous uveitis, the formation of adhesions to the IOL is likely to be retarded.[22–24] It has been suggested that heparin-surface-modified models provide an impressive cell-free IOL surface and greater protection from inflammatory complications as with unmodified lenses.[25] On the other hand, if cellular adhesion is reduced by implanting heparin-surface-modified lenses, the IOL will be clearer and visual acuity enhanced.[26] A recent report has shown that mechanical irritation during the implantation procedure destroys the heparin layer on PMMA IOLs in the grasp area. Clinical consequences are not yet known.[27]

Limited information is available regarding foldable IOL implantation in patients with chronic uveitis. PMMA is the most commonly used intraocular lens material. It has proved to be inert and stable, and its manufacture has been optimized over decades.[28] Materials like silicone and hydrogel have been progressively accepted for intraocular implants in humans. New technology applied to PMMA lenses has enabled the development of a new generation of acrylic foldable lenses for small incision surgery.

Silicone lenses have displayed greater inflammatory reaction after ECCE in uveitic patients when compared with other types of lenses (PMMA, Heparin-modified, hydrogel).[29] After phacoemulsification procedures, a number of complications have been described such as intense inflammatory reactions in the anterior chamber, the total closure of the capsulorhexis[30] and an increase in posterior capsule opacification when compared with PMMA implants.

Acrylic lenses (PMMA foldable lenses) are available for small incision surgery. The intraocular behavior of this material is known and is perhaps the best of all foldable intraocular lenses at present. We lack information about its implantation in patients with uveitis, but this is one of the coming challenges for these IOLs.

In patients with only one functional eye, the surgeon may consider not implanting an IOL.

■ Postoperative Treatment

Postoperative care should include the maintenance of prior medications required for the control of the disorder with gradual reduction. Periocular injections of Triamcinolone are routinely used after phacoemulsification procedures (Trigon Depot R 0.5 ml).

Suggested Postoperative Medications:
1. The topical steroid treatment should be continued with Prednisolone 1%, eight times a day for the first week, to be gradually decreased over a period of months.
2. Diclofenac, four times a day for 2 weeks.
3. Tropicamide 1% four times a day for 4 weeks.
4. If the IOP is elevated, beta blockers, dorzolamide, or systemic acetazolamide are used.
5. Oral Prednisone 1 mg/kg/day for 2 weeks, tapering it down for another 2 weeks for a total of one month.

Persistent uncontrolled glaucoma will require filtration surgery with the use of Mitomycin C 0.02% applied for 2 minutes under the scleral flap.[31] Pupillary membranes after cataract surgery can be removed by pars plana vitrectomy techniques.[32]

Cystoid macular edema is the most serious postoperative complication in patients with chronic uveitis who undergo cataract extraction. This complication occurs in 50% of the cases and is present in 80% of eyes with less than 20/40 of postoperative visual acuity.[33,34] Cystoid macular edema may be treated with oral acetazolamide, a topical nonsteroidal anti-inflammatory agent, or topical, periocular injections, and systemic steroids.

■ Cataract Surgery in Specific Cases of Uveitis

Phacoemulsifiction in Fuchs' Heterochromic Cyclitis

The uveitis associated with Fuchs' Heterochromic Cyclitis (FHC) tends to be chronic and of low intensity. Posterior synechiae are rarely formed and the patients are usually unaware of the problem until the first complication arises cataracts or vitreous opacities.[35] Posterior subcapsular cataract is the most commonly seen complication in these patients.[36]

The implantation of IOLs in patients with FHC is generally satisfactory with good visual outcome. Some authors have reported the use of heparin-surface modified lenses for all patients with FHC in whom implantation is indicated.[37]

Fuchs' Heterochromic Cyclitis patients have few postoperative complications although some isolated cases of vitreitis, hyphema, increase of intraocular pressure, and cyclitic membrane formation have been reported.[38] Posterior capsule pacification has been described in 8 to 20% of the patients. The problem with greatest visual significance is the development of glaucoma which appear in approximately 10% (3 to 35%) of the patients, and up to 70% of them may require filtration surgery.[35]

Some risk factors have been identified in these patients. If glaucoma was present preoperatively, it may worsen postoperatively. In cases of severe iris atrophy, the risk of postoperative uveitis appears to be higher. When rubeosis iridis is present and hemorrhage occurs during surgery, the risk of both postoperative uveitis and glaucoma is higher.

Sarcoidosis

Sarcoidosis is a systemic granulomatous disorder of unknown etiology, presenting with bilateral hilar adenopathy, pulmonary infiltration and, eye involvement. Ocular lesions occur in approximately 25 to 50% of patients with systemic sarcoidosis.[39] In patients with ocular sarcoidosis, chronic granulomatous panuveitis is the most common manifestation.[40] Cataract formation is a frequent complication of sarcoidosis.

Phacoemulsification has been performed with good results in a series of patients.[41] Intraoperative miosis is the rule and sphincterotomies or other mechanical techniques are commonly necessary.

Single piece PMMA are the IOLs of choice. Silicone lenses have also been used with good results. Most frequent postoperative visual complications include chronic posterior uveitis and cystoid macular edema; glaucoma; and posterior capsule opacification (50%).

Syphilis

Patients diagnosed with syphilitic uveitis must receive prior treatment with antibiotics for their illness, and the cases which have an important postoperative reaction tend to remit with topical steroid treatment. Treponemic infection often tends to persist in spite of antibiotic treatment.[42]

Pars Planitis

Inflammation in patients with pars planitis (PP) is initially limited to the posterior segment. A slight iridocyclitic reaction is present in some cases; synechiae are thus rare and glaucoma is an exception.[43] Cataracts develop in 40% of the patients. The lens opacity starts as diffuse posterior subcapsular areas.

Vision improves after cataract extraction and 50% obtain 20/40 vision or better. Few studies report phacoemulsification techniques in patients with pars planitis. Pars planitis does not seem to increase the risk of complications in routine cataract surgery. Often, a low degree of postoperative inflammation persists with an accumulation of debris and membranes on the back surface of the IOL and on the posterior capsule. These membranes have been described to surround the IOL in patients with PP. High energy YAG laser spots might be needed. These membranes tend to return and can be controlled with subconjunctival and frequent topical steroids.[44,45]

Chronic Juvenile Arthritis (CJA)

Patients are usually young females affected by monoarticular or pauci-articular juvenile rheumatoid arthritis with positive test for antinuclear antibodies and HLA DR5.

Complications include band keratopathy, posterior synechiae, hypotony, glaucoma, and cataracts. Most of the patients develop these complications in the first decade of life. Children who develop media opacity may have an associated amblyopia along with their inflammatory problems.

The average age at the time of the operation varies between series from 10 to 19 years[46] but children as young as 4 years old may need surgery as well.

Patients with CJA have exacerbation of the uveitic process after cataract surgery. Surgery on these patients involves serious intraoperative complications, with vitreous loss and retained cortical material in good percentage of patients. Vision of 20/200 or worse is found in up to 60% of the cases.[47] Performing an anterior and mid-portion vitrectomy is recommended by some authors with apparently good results.[48]

Uveitis associated with CJA is at present a contraindication for IOL implantation. Phacoemulsification without IOL implantation, whether associated or not with a pars plana vitrectomy, is the preferred technique.

The most common postoperative complications are glaucoma, hypotony and macular edema.[49]

Standard cataract surgery is recommended if the eye has no signs of vitreitis nor vitreous opacities. Should these be present a combined procedure is then suggested.

Behcet's Disease, Vogt-Koyanagi-Harada, and Multifocal Chorioretinitis

There are few reports on cataract surgery or phacoemulsification in patients with Behcet's disease, Vogt-Koyanagi-Harada, and multifocal chorioretinitis (Figs. 8–3 and 8–4).

The incidence of phthisis bulbi and hypotony has been reported to decrease from 25% to 2% when limited vitrectomy was performed in combination with cataract extrac-

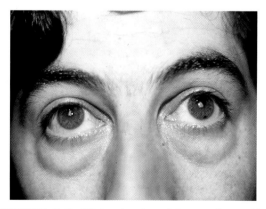

FIGURE 8–3. Bilateral cataract in a patient with Behcet's disease with neurological manifestation. Light perception vision as a result of retinal vasculitis and anterior segment inflammation. It is difficult to estimate the potential vision in these cases.

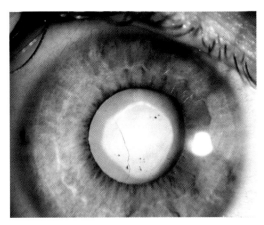

FIGURE 8–4. Total cataract in a patient with Behcet's disease. Anterior capsular fibrosis is frequent and capsulorhexis very difficult.

tion.[50] It is not clear, however, whether vitrectomy combined with cataract extraction can alter the course of inflammation. Visual prognosis is significantly worse in eyes with Behcet's disease than other types of idiopathic uveitis because of the severe posterior segment complications, particularly optic atrophy.[51]

Phacoemulsification or ECCE and vitrectomy in multifocal chorioretinitis with panuveitis has little therapeutic benefit. Surgical treatment shows no obvious effect on the intensity or frequency of uveitis relapse. When an IOL is implanted, a visual improvement of one or two lines can be expected, but visual acuity returns to preoperative values within 6 months. Multifocal chorioretinitis remains poorly understood in terms of its etiology and suitable treatment.[52]

Other Forms of Uveitis

Patients with Herpes Zoster uveitis have few complications after an IOL implantation. Visual acuity is better than 20/40 in 90% of the cases. In 18% of these cases a chronic uveitis persists.[53]

Anterior forms of idiopathic uveitis have favorable prognosis with excellent functional visual recovery. The same does not occur when the idiopathic uveitis involves the posterior segment or is a panuveitis.

Other forms of uveitis that can benefit from IOL implantation with a good visual prognosis include ankylosing spondylitis, Crohn's disease, and toxoplasmosis.[54]

■ Tips and Pearls

1. Control of the preoperative inflammatory state is mandatory. A minimum of 3 months of quiescence is necessary before surgery is indicated. Topical, periocular, and systemic medications can be used for this purpose.
2. It will require a delicate surgery, maximum mydriasis, and the use of viscoelastic material.
3. Careful cortical removal and posterior capsular polishing are important steps to prevent or delay posterior capsular opacification frequently found in these patients. An anterior vitrectomy can be performed should vitreous opacities be present at the time of surgery.
4. Intraocular lenses can be implanted in the majority of uveitic patients. Until further studies are done in this area, implantation of heparin-coated PMMA or acrylic lenses are at present, the best approach.
5. The postoperative control of inflammation is extremely important in these patients since the complications associated with it may be severe. Complications associated with postoperative elevations of intraocular pressure can be as important.
6. Chronic juvenile arthritis tends to exacerbate the uveitis after cataract surgery. In these patients, a careful decision for IOL implantation must be made. At present, is not recommended.
7. In children, the surgery will be of no value unless intensive treatment for amblyopia is performed immediately after the surgery.

REFERENCES

1. Tabbara KF, Chavis PS. Cataract extraction in patients with chronic posterior uveitis. Int Ophthalmol Clin 1995;35:121–131.
2. Alio JL, Chipont E, Sayans JA. Postoperative inflammation following non-complicated extracapsular sur-

gery with intraocular lens implantation: Sulcus vs in the bag implantation. J Cataract Refract Surg 1996;22:775–779.
3. Alio JL, Claramonte P, Ruiz Moreno JM, Palomares JM. Frequency of the posterior opacification with Nd-YAG capsulotomy related to inflammatory complications in extracapsular cataract surgery. Book of the Third International Symposium on Ocular Inflammation, Fukuoka, Japan; 1994:221.
4. Mondino BJ, Rao H. Effect of intraocular lenses on complacent levels in human serum. Acta Ophthalmol 1983;61:76–94.
5. Kaplan HJ, Discussion of Foster CS, Fong LP, Singh G. Cataract surgery and intraocular lens implantation in patients with uveitis. Ophthalmology 1989;96:287–288.
6. Foster CS. Vitrectomy in the management of uveitis (guest editorial). Ophthalmology 1988;95:1011–1012.
7. Chipont E, Espana E, Munoz G, Sanchez S, Diaz M. Penetration intraocular de la ciclosporina A en pacientes con uveitis. Arch Soc Esp Oftalmol 1995; 68:517–524.
8. Foster CS and Barrett F. Cataract development and cataract surgery in patients with juvenile rheumatoid arthritis-associated iridocyclitis. Ophthalmology 1993, 100(6): 809–817.
9. Dangel ME, Stark WJ, Michels RG. Surgical management of cataracts associated with chronic uveitis. Ophthalmic Surg 1983;14:145–149.
10. Diamond JG, Kaplan HJ. Lensectomy and vitrectomy for complicated cataract secondary to uveitis. Arch Ophthalmol 1978;95:1798–1804.
11. Girard LJ, Rodriguez J, Mailman ML, Romano TJ. Cataract and uveitis management by pars plana lensectomy and vitrectomy by ultrasonic fragmentation. Retina 1985;5:107–114.
12. Chipont E, Martinez JJ. Intrastomal corneal suture for small incision cataract surgery. J Cataract Refract Surg 1996;22:671–675.
13. Koening SB, Han DP, Mieler WF, Abrams GW, Jaffe GJ, Burgon TC. Combined phacoemulsification and pars plana vitrectomy. Arch Ophthalmol 1990;108: 362–364.
14. MacKool RJ. Pars plana vitrectomy and posterior chamber intraocular lens implantation in diabetic patients. Ophthalmology 1989;96:1679–1680.
15. Nobe JR, Kokoris D, Diddie KR. Lensectomy—vitrectomy in chronic uveitis. Retina 1983;3:71–76.
16. Nolthenius PA, Deutman AF. Surgical treatment of the complications of chronic uveitis. Ophthalmologica. 1983;186:11–16.
17. Lichter PR. Intraocular lenses in uveitis patients (editorial). Ophthalmology 1980;96:279–280.
18. Hooper PL, Rao NA, Smith RE. Cataract extraction in uveitis patients Surv Ophthalmol 1990;35:120–143.
19. Foster CS, Fong LP, Singh G. Cataract surgery and intraocular lens implantation in patients with uveitis. Ophthalmology 1989;96:281–287.
20. Lowenstein A, Bracha R, Lazar M. Intraocular lens implantation in an eye with Behcet's uveitis. J Cataract Refr Surg 1991;17:95–97.
21. Foster CS, Fong LP, Singh G. Cataract Surgery and intraocular lens implantation in patients with uveitis. Ophthalmology 1989;96P:281–287.
22. Ygge J, Wenzel M, Philipson B. Cellular reactions on heparin surface-modified versus regular PMMA lenses during the first postoperative month. Ophthalmology 1990;97:1216–1223.
23. Miyake K, Maekubo K. Comparison of heparin surface modified and ordinary PCLS: a Japanese study. European J Implant Refract Surg 1991;3:95–97.
24. Borgioli M, Coster DJ, Fan RFT. Effect of heparin surface modification on polymethylmethacrylate intraocular lenses on signs of postoperative inflammation after extracapsular cataract extraction. Ophthalmology 1992;99:1248–1255.
25. Percival SPB, Pai V. Heparin-modified lenses for eyes at risk for breakdown of the blood-aqueous barrier during cataract surgery. J Cataract Refr Surg 1993;19: 760–765.
26. Jones NP. Extracapsular cataract surgery with an without intraocular lens implantation in Fuchs' heterochronic uveitis. Am J Ophthalmol 1989;108: 310–314.
27. Dick B, Kohnen T, Jacobi KW. Alterations of heparin coating on intraocular lenses caused by implantation instruments. Klin Moatsbl Augenheilkd 1995;206 (6):460–466.
28. Drews, RC Lens implantation lessons learned from the first million. Trans Ophthalmol Soc UK 1982; 102:505–509.
29. Alio JL, Sayans J, Chipont E. Laser flare-cell measurement of inflammation after uneventful extracapsular cataract extraction and intraocular lens implantation. J Cataract Refract Surg 1996;22:775–779.
30. Martinez JJ, Artola A, Chipont E. Total anterior capsule closure after silicone intraocular lens implantation. J Cataract Refract Surg 1996;22:269–271.
31. Ruiz Moreno JM, Alio JL, Alcazar A, Artola A, Lozano M. Etude de la toxicite sur lendothelium cormeen de la Mitomycine C injectee dans la chambre anterieur. Ophthalmologie 1994;8:45–49.
32. Puig-Llano M, Irvine AR, Stone RD. Pupillary membrane excision and anterior vitrectomy in eyes after uveitis. Am J Ophthalmol 1979;87:533–535.
33. Nussemblatt RB, Kaufman SC, Palestine AG. Macular thickening and visual acuity: measurement in patients with cystoid macular edema. Ophthalmology 1987;94: 1134–1139.
34. Palestine AG, Alter GJ, Chan CC. Laser interferometry and visual prognosis in uveitis. Ophthalmology 1985;92:1567–1569.
35. Liesegang TJ. Clinical features and prognosis in Fuchs' uveitis syndrome. Arch Ophthalmol 1982;100: 1622–1626.
36. Franceschetti A. Heterochromic Cyclitis (Fuchs' syndrome). Am J Opthalmol 1955;39:50–58.
37. Jones NP. Cataract surgery using heparin surface modified intraocular lenses in Fuchs' heterochromic uveitis. Ophthalmic Surg 1995;26:49–52.
38. Mills KB, Rosen ES. Intraocular lens implantation following cataract extraction in Fuchs' heterochromic uveitis. Ophthalmol Surg 1982;13:467.

39. Rothova A, Albersts C, Glasius E. Risk factors for ocular sarcoidosis. Doc opthalmol 1989;72:287–408.
40. James DG, Neville E, Langley DA. Ocular sarcoidosis. Trans Ophthalmol Soc UK 1976;96:133–139.
41. Jabs DA, Johns CJ. Ocular involvement in chronic sarcoidosis. Am J Ophthalmol 1986;102:297–301.
42. Ryan SJ, Hardy PH, Hardy JM, Oppennheimer GH. Persistence of virulent treponema pallidum despite penicillin therapy in congenital syphilis. Am J Opthalmol 1972;2:77–83.
43. Smith RE, Godfrey WA, Kimura SJ. Complications of chronic cyclitis. Am J Ophthalmo 1976;82:277–282.
44. Michelson JB, Friedlander MH, Nozik RA. Lens implant surgery in pars planitis. Ophthalmology 1990; 97:1023–1026.
45. Wolter JR. Cytopathology of intraocular lens implantation. Ophthalmology 1985;92:135–142.
46. Pivetti-Pezzi P, Moncada A, Torce MC, Santillo C. Causes of reduced visual acuity on long term follow up after cataract extraction in patients with uveitis and juvenile rheumatoid arthritis. Am J Opthalmol 1993;115(6): 826–827.
47. Key SN III, Kimura SJ. Iridocyclitis associated with Juvenile Rheumatoid Arthritis. Am J Ophthalmol 1975; 80:425.
48. Michelson JB, Nozik RA, Smith RA. Uveitis Surgery. In Duanes's Clinical Ophthalmology 4th ed. Philadelphia: J.B. Lippincott Company, 1991.
49. Wolf MD, Lichter PR, Ragsdale CG. Prognosis factors in the uveitis of Juvenile Rheumatoid Arthritis. Ophthalmology 1987;94:1242–1248.
50. Kanski JJ, Shun-Shin GA. Systemic uveitis syndrome in childhood; an analysis of 340 cases. Ophthalmology 1984;91:1247–1252.
51. Ciftci OU, Ozdemir, O. Cataract extraction comparative study of ocular Behcet's disease and idiopathic uveitis. Ophthalmologuica 1995;209:270–274.
52. Nolle B, Eckart C. Vitrectomy in multifocal chorioretinitis. Ger J Ophthalmol 1993;2(1):14–19.
53. Marsh RJ, Copper M. Ocular surgery in ophthalmic zoster. Eye 1989;3:313–317.
54. Foster RE, Lowder CY, Meisler DM, Zakov ZN. Extracapsular cataract extraction and posterior chamber intraocular lens implantation in uveitis patients. Ophthalmology 1992;99:1234–1241.

9

Phacoemulsification in a Previous Functioning Glaucoma Surgery

LUIS W. LU

The development of cataracts or the progression of a previous lens opacity is one of the most common complications following a filtering procedure, with a reported incidence between 15 and 42 % following trabeculectomy.[1-4]

Several factors may play a role in cataract formation such as direct trauma to the lens, hypotony, shallowing or flattening of the anterior chamber with lens-cornea touch, and changes in the aqueous humor dynamics. The percentage of bleb failure after cataract extraction in patients with previous functioning filtering surgery ranges from 0 to more than 50%.[5-8] The high rate of bleb failure poses a challenge to the surgeon.

Cataract extraction in a patient with previous glaucoma surgery includes those patients with previous iridectomy, cyclodyalisis, trabeculotomy, tube/shunt, and filtering surgeries as trabeculectomy, iridencleisis, Scheie procedure, sclerostomy with the Holmium laser, etc. This chapter refers to cataract surgery in the presence of a functioning filtering bleb and a controlled glaucoma (Fig. 9–1).

The main concern in these patients is the long-term control of the intraocular pressure after a successful cataract surgery. The questions in this particular situation will be: the preoperative considerations; location of the incision; management of posterior synechias and small pupil; special considerations during cataract surgery, and the postoperative management.

In those patients without a functioning bleb, the preoperative assessment of the cataract and the type and degree of damage from the glaucoma will determine the management of these two conditions with basically three options: a combined cataract and glaucoma surgery, cataract surgery alone, or the two-stage surgery with the filter first and the cataract surgery later. The first option is described in chapter 10.

■ Preoperative Considerations

After a successful glaucoma filtering procedure, it should be possible to reduce glaucoma medications including the elimination of miotics. The disadvantages of this second stage cataract procedure will be the possible loss of the long-term control of the intraocular pressure and the technical difficulty in the presence of a bleb.

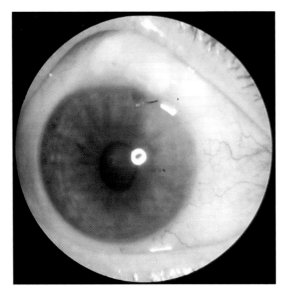

FIGURE 9–1. Presence of a functioning bleb and cataract.

Evaluation of the bleb function is important. The preoperative intraocular pressure will help decide if an internal revision of the bleb will be required. Gonioscopy can determine the patency of the sclerostomy opening. Evaluation of the glaucomatous cupping will inform the surgeon if the optic nerve will be able to survive an immediate postoperative spike in intraocular pressure and the precautions that have to be taken.

The preoperative evaluation will include the description of the type of cataract present to determine in advance the technique of phacoemulsification to be utilized; preoperative measurement of the maximum pupil dilation that might suggest the intraoperative use of techniques of pupillary dilation; the keratometry; and whenever possible, the preoperative topography to help us decide if an astigmatic surgery combined with the cataract extraction will be required. In patients with advanced glaucomatous damage, the patient should have a clear understanding of the condition of the eye to prevent false expectations.

Timing is very important; wait as long as possible after a successful glaucoma surgery, preferably a minimum of 12 months. Mature filtration blebs that have been established for more than 1 year are probably more resistant to the insult arising from the additional intraocular surgery than the less mature ones.[9] Most filtering bleb failures occur within the first year after trabeculectomy. If the patient requires the surgery earlier, the surgeon must take the necessary precautions.

Remember not to apply any external manual compression, superpinky, or Honan balloon prior to the surgery because the external pressure may cause compression of the bleb and intraocular pressure spike which can cause further damage.

■ Location of the Incision

The surgeon should plan the type of incision in advance. The smaller the incision the less inflammation. Certainly a clear corneal incision will be indicated since this minimizes conjunctival manipulation. Although a superiorly located incision adjacent to the bleb may provide easiest access to the phacoemulsification tip (Fig. 9–2), as with an incision anterior to the bleb (Fig. 9–3), it may prove to be a technically more difficult phacoemulsification procedure while trying to avoid the bleb. An increase of a preoperative against-the-rule astigmatism is also expected from these inci-

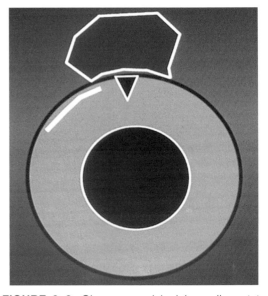

FIGURE 9–2. Clear corneal incision adjacent to the bleb.

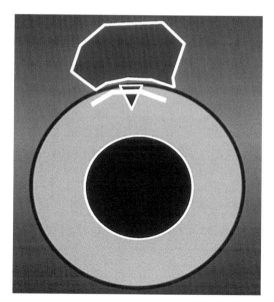

FIGURE 9–3. Clear corneal incision anterior to the bleb.

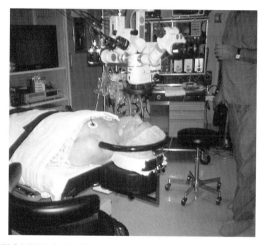

FIGURE 9–5. Room preparation for temporal approach surgery.

sions, as well as possibly more endothelial damage from the superiorly located incision.[11]

A temporal or infero-temporal clear corneal incision approach 90 degrees away from the bleb might be the incision of choice. A scleral tunnel incision from the temporal side is not contraindicated (Fig. 9–4). The surgeon should be familiar with the techniques and ergonomics of this temporal approach (Fig. 9–5).

■ Management of Posterior Synechias and Small Pupil

Management of the small pupil during surgery, certainly can be encountered when performing cataract surgery in the presence of a previous glaucoma surgery. The small pupil may be secondary to posterior synechia, diabetes, or pseudoexfoliation, or previous long-term use of miotics.

Our protocol for the dilation of these patients includes the use of Tropicamide 1% and Cyclopentolate 1% every 5 minutes times three, and a drop of Phenylephrine 2.5% once or twice unless contraindicated, starting 90 minutes prior to the scheduled surgery.

A pupil dilation of 5 mm should be sufficient for a routine phacoemulsification procedure. For patients with pseudoexfoliation, with dense cataracts and whenever the surgeon requires to have a larger pupil diameter, a mechanical dilation has to be considered. The more intraocular manipulations performed, the more postoperative inflammation will be induced, with increased possibility of bleb failure.

Sphinterotomies, sphinterectomy, iridectomy, bimanual iris stretching techniques, the Beehler pupil dilator, different self-retaining iris retractors, and the pupil expanders are used as surgeon preference for the mechanical pupillary dilation. Along with these intraoperative maneuvers such as avoiding excessive iris manipulation, addition of epinephrine in the bottle of infusion, sweeping and releasing synechia, pupillary expansion with viscoelastics, and striping of a peripupillary membrane are performed when needed.

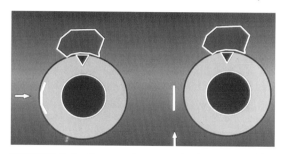

FIGURE 9–4. Temporal approach clear corneal incision.

Special Considerations During Cataract Surgery

There are many causes for filtering bleb failure following cataract surgery. Inadvertent bleb trauma may occur during surgery. Prolonged hypotony during the procedure may cause adherence of the bleb walls and inflammatory components in the aqueous may seal the bleb. Remnants of lens material or capsule can block the opening of the fistula.

A clear corneal incision should be the surgeon's preference, because it minimizes the postoperative inflammatory reaction. In regard to the location of the incision, it is preferable to stay away from the bleb. The location may also be determined by the preoperative astigmatism and convenience for the surgeon as well.

Capsulorhexis is done under viscoelastic material with removal of the excised capsule preventing blockage of the sclerostomy by any capsular remnant. Anterior cleavage hydrodissection and nucleus rotation are performed as the usual manner, except in the presence of pseudoexfoliation or cases of zonular dehiscence where appropriate precautions have to be taken.

Direct trauma to the bleb is avoided. During the clear corneal incision, the use of scleral fixation devices is also avoided (Fig. 9–6). During the procedure, moving the corneal incision towards the infero-temporal quadrant minimizes manipulation of the bleb while using a second instrument through a paracentesis port.

Care is taken during phacoemulsification and irrigation-aspiration to maintain the fistula free of nuclear and cortical fragments. Attention to the anterior chamber depth and infusion bottle height are important, since more dynamic changes in the anterior segment will be observed, as compared with the routine phacoemulsification procedure (Figs. 9–7 and 9–8). Careful capsular polishing is performed under viscoelastic, preferably under sodium hyaluronate which can be easily removed after the intraocular lens implantation.

The personal preference is to utilize an acrylic foldable lens and to have a incision size of 3.2 mm or less (Fig. 9–9).

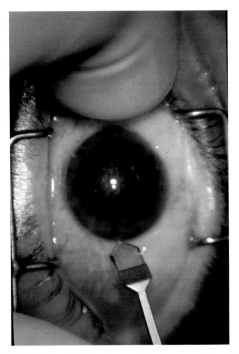

FIGURE 9–6. Performing a clear corneal incision without a fixation device.

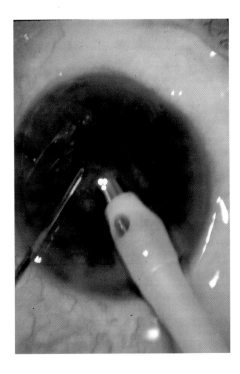

FIGURE 9–7. Phacoemulsification.

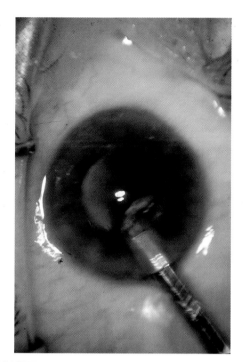

FIGURE 9–8. Irrigation and aspiration.

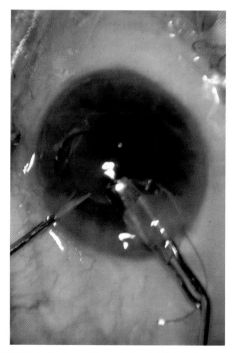

FIGURE 9–9. Insertion of the foldable intraocular lens without a ring fixation device.

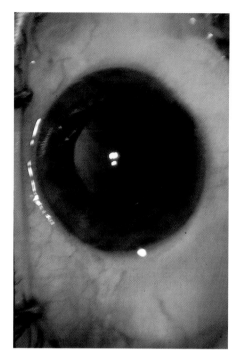

FIGURE 9–10. Confirming the bleb function.

The viscoelastic material is removed and the bleb function confirmed, by filling the anterior chamber with balanced salt solution (Fig. 9–10). If bleb formation is not noticed, an internal revision of the bleb has to be performed. The anterior chamber is again filled with sufficient viscoelastic material, a cyclodialysis spatula is inserted through the wound or a paracentesis and is passed through the sclerostomy and under the bleb (Fig. 9–11). With circular movements, the spatula is used to open the scleral flap and dissect the con-

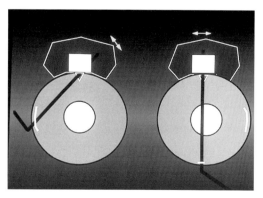

FIGURE 9–11. Internal bleb revision.

junctiva around the bleb in an arc-like fashion.[12] Sometimes a vigorous dissection is required.[11] If the sclerostomy opening is not found, a four-mirror goniolens is utilized. A remaining cortical or capsular material can be drained away through the flapless sclerostomy with this maneuver. It can also be considered done in eyes with previous filtration surgery and borderline outflow through the sclerostomy, preventing hypofunction of the bleb.

Internal bleb revision has been advocated to be performed routinely in all patients with previous filter whenever the preoperative pressure is 6 mmHg or more to promote preservation of the filtering bleb.[9]

Removal of the viscoelastic material is important, and performed as suggested by Assia for a minimum of 20 to 25 seconds of irrigation and aspiration in all four quadrants and from under the intraocular lens, preventing a postoperative rise in intraocular pressure.[10]

The procedure does not necessarily have to be sutureless, if the surgeon considers that digital massage may be necessary during the postoperative period. In these cases a crossed 10–0 nylon or radial sutures, are applied prior to the removal of the viscoelastic material and tightened after the removal is completed and the anterior chamber formed. The suture allows the patients to use digital pressure without the risk of wound dehiscence.

Application of topical mitomycin to the bleb at the time of cataract surgery has been studied with early encouraging results.[11] Applied at the same concentration and time as in trabeculectomy with a mitomycin-soaked pledget, copious irrigation with balanced salt solution is performed after. The other alternative will be the use of topical 5 FU, 50 mg/ml for 5 minutes.

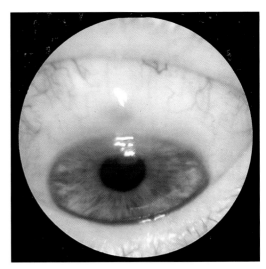

FIGURE 9–12. Postoperative photograph of an eye postphacoemulsification through a clear corneal incision in the presence of a functioning filtering bleb.

use of topical steroids with Prednisolone phosphate 1% every hour or two while the patient is awake is required, and gradually tapering it over a 1 to 2 month period.

Topical antibiotic is given four times a day for 2 weeks. The use of cycloplegics may be considered as a bedtime drop. Digital massage and subconjunctival injection of 5-FU may be considered as after a trabeculectomy procedure.

We must expect some loss of long-term intraocular pressure control after cataract surgery which may be able to be prevented. Closed follow up during the postoperative period is very important, and additional antiglaucomatous medications might be required (Fig. 9–12).

■ Tips and Pearls

1. Perform a careful preoperative functional evaluation of the previous filtering procedure.
2. Determine if mechanical dilation will be required at the time of cataract surgery, and be prepared.
3. Wait as long as possible after the functioning filter surgery, for the cataract procedure.

■ The Postoperative Management

Early postoperative intraocular pressure spikes are frequently observed after cataract surgery in glaucomatous eyes, and considerable fluctuations in pressure can occur during the first postoperative month.[13–15]

The preoperative antiglaucomatous medications if any, must be continued. Vigorous

4. Temporal clear corneal approach is preferred.
5. Attention to the anterior chamber depth and infusion bottle height.
6. Stay away from the bleb as possible.
7. The smaller the incision the better.
8. Check for bleb function at the end of the procedure. If there are any doubts, consider internal bleb revision or topical mitomycin over the bleb.
9. Apply a suture if digital massage is a consideration for the postoperative period.
10. Vigorous use of steroids in the postoperative period is required.
11. Consider 5-FU injections if any signs of postoperative bleb failure.

REFERENCES

1. Keroub C, Hyams SW, Rath E. Study of cataract formation following trabeculectomy. Glaucoma 1984; 6: 117.
2. Salmon JF. The role of trabeculectomy in the treatment of advanced chronic angle closure glaucoma. J Glaucoma 1993;2:4.
3. Popovic V, Sjostrand J. Long term outcome following trabeculectomy: I. Retrospective analysis of IOP regulation and cataract formation. Acta Ophthalmol (Copenh) 1991;69:299–304.
4. Deschartes F, Labrune PA, Clavel D, Gillibert A. Resultant a long terme de la trabeculectomie. J Fr Ophthalmol 1985;8:705–710.
5. Kass MA. Cataract extraction in an eye with a filtering bleb. Ophthalmology 1982;89:871–874.
6. Frankelson EN, Shaffer RN. The management of coexisting cataract and glaucoma. Can J Ophthalmol 1974;9:298–301.
7. Balaglou P, Matta C, Asdourian K. Cataract extraction after filtering operations. Arch Ophthalmol 1972;88: 12–15.
8. Brooks AM, Gillies WA. The effect of cataract extraction with implant in glaucomatous eyes. Aus N Z J Ophthalmol (Aus) 1992;20(3):235–238.
9. Nasahara N, Sibayan S, Montenegro M, Simmons RB, Smith TJ. Corneal incision phacoemulsification and internal bleb revision. Ophthal Surg Lasers 1996;27: 361–366.
10. Assia EI, Castaneda VE, Legler UF, et al. Studies on cataract surgery and intraocular lenses at the center for intraocular lens research. Ophtahlmol Clin North Am 1991;4:251–266.
11. Shingleton BJ (ed). Surgical Management of Coexisting Cataract and Glaucoma. (CD). Boston: Ophthalmology Interactive; 1996.
12. Sofinski SJ, Thomas JV, Simmons RJ. Filtering bleb revision technique. In: Thomas JV (ed). Glaucoma Surgery. St. Louis: Mosby; 1992;77.
13. Seah SK, Jap A, Prata JA, Baerveldt G, Lee PP, et al. Cataract surgery after trabeculectomy. Ophthal Surg Lasers 1996;27:587–594.
14. McGuigan LJ, Gottsch J, Stark WJ, et al. Extracapsular cataract extraction and posterior chamber lens implantation in eyes with pre-existing glaucoma. Arch Ophthalmol 1986;104:1301–1308.
15. Atagi K, Araie M, Ando K, et al. Intraocular lens implantation after glaucoma filtering surgery- time course of changes in intraocular pressure control and filtering blebs. Nippon Ganka Gakkai Zasshi (Japan) 1992;96:1274–1281.

10

Phacoemulsification in Combined Cataract and Glaucoma Surgery

ALAN S. CRANDALL

At the present time there are many options available for the treatment of concomitant glaucoma and cataract.[1-13] The gold standard remains a trabeculectomy followed at a later date (3–6 months) by a cataract extraction. The advantage of this approach is that frequently the pupil may return to normal and facilitate the cataract extraction. However, there is the delay in visual recovery, there is the expense of two surgeries, and while many feel there is overall better control of glaucoma, some filters will fail after cataract extraction.

Patients with well controlled glaucoma and a healthy optic nerve may benefit from phacoemulsification of the cataract with implantation of a posterior chamber lens since this group will likely have a 3 to 4 mm pressure drop that is consistent at 1 year. One may consider a cataract extraction with the use of endophotocoagulation of the ciliary processes. This relatively new procedure, however, has not undergone any controlled studies and no long-term data is available. The pressure may take time to reduce and there is frequently inflammation from the laser process.

Multiple studies have shown the efficacy of combined phacoemulsification and trabeculectomy.[1-3,5,14-20] Many surgeons now favor an approach that consists of a temporal clear corneal cataract extraction with foldable intraocular lens followed by a superior trabeculectomy.[10,21] This is an approach that I use if there is poor exposure superiorly since this is my standard cataract extraction. However, if there is easy access superiorly, I will do a standard single site combined phacoemulsification with trabeculectomy usually with adjunctive anti-metabolite.[6-10,22-25]

■ Preoperative

Indications for combined procedures involve many factors. These should include a preoperative evaluation of the visual disability caused by the cataract, the state of the optic nerve, and hence, the need to control pressure in patients with advanced glaucoma or split fixation. The decision may also include the intolerance or noncompliance with medications.

■ Surgical Technique

Anesthesia

Combined procedures are now done under topical medications. An IV is started and patients receive 0.5 to 1.0 mg of Versed. They may receive 50 μg of Fentanyl. Prior to entering the operating room, three sets of drops (two drops) of 0.75% Bupivicaine (Marcaine [R]) are given. Following the prep, the patient will receive two more drops. After draping and the lid speculum is placed, a small Weck-cel sponge soaked in Marcaine is placed on the superior conjunctiva for 1 to 2 minutes.

A conjunctival limbal peritomy[26] is made with blunt Wescott scissors, creating a fornix-based conjunctival flap. This is measured to be 6 mm long, a small amount (0.5 mm) of the limbal conjunctiva remains which facilitates the closure and preserves the limbal palisades (Fig. 10–1).

A tenonectomy is no longer performed. Hemostasis is obtained by the wet-field cautery. This tends to be the only portion of the procedure that the patients feel. A diamond knife is used to fashion two partial-depth (0.3 mm) radial incisions, these are 4.0 mm apart and extend 2.0 mm posterior to the limbus. The radial incisions are then connected posteriorly (Fig. 10–2). A trabeculectomy flap is shelved anteriorly a 1/2 scleral thickness depth with a diamond crescent blade.

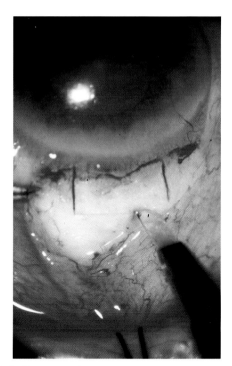

FIGURE 10–2. Delineating the trabeculectomy flap.

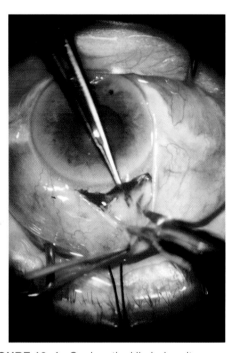

FIGURE 10–1. Conjunctival limbal peritomy.

Prior to entering the eye, a sponge soaked in 0.2 mg/ml Mitomycin-C is placed in the sclera and allowed to sit with contact to Tenon's capsule for 2.5 minutes (up to 4 minutes). Care is taken not to expose the conjunctival edge that will be used for closure, to the mitomycin.

The sac is then irrigated with a balanced salt solution (BSS). A stab incision is made for the second instrument through clear cornea. Then 0.3 cc of unpreserved 1% Lidocaine is injected into the anterior chamber. Aqueous is exchanged for viscoelastic and the eye is entered with a keratome through the trabeculectomy flap (Fig. 10–3).

At this point the iris must be dealt with.[27-31] Frequently these patients have small pupils that need to be enlarged. Several studies have shown that the main indicator for complications is a small pupil, followed by pseudoexfoliation. Most pupils can be enlarged simply by a slow stretching maneuver with two hooks. A Beehler pupil dilator (Moria instruments, Antony, France), can also give a controlled, slow pupil enlargement. If this

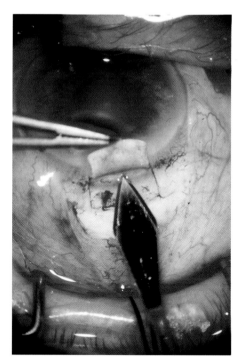

FIGURE 10–3. The eye is entered with the keratome.

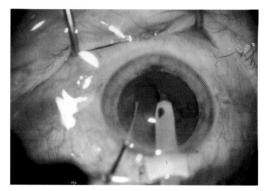

FIGURE 10–4. The nucleus is emulsified.

fails, multiple (6-8) small sphincterotomies as described by I. Howard Fine[30] will suffice.

The Grieshaber iris hooks can be used as well. Care must be taken to enter as close to the iris as possible to eliminate problems with the phacoemulsification. A Graether pupil expander is another elegant method to enlarge the pupil.

Following pupillary enlargement, a Utrata forceps is used to perform a capsulorhexis, a 5.0 to 5.5 central capsulotomy is preferred. The lens is then hydrodissected and hydrodelineated with a syringe of BSS. I prefer a 25 or 27 gauge cannula.

The nucleus is then emulsified. My preferred technique is to groove centrally, usually with a Kelman-tip, 60% power, 30 mmHg of vacuum, and 14 cc/min of aspiration flow rate (Alcon 20,000 unit) (Fig. 10–4). The nucleus is rotated 180 degrees to facilitate central grooving, and it is then hemisected. The power of the phaco unit is dropped to 50%, vacuum increased to around 300 mmHg and aspiration flow rate increased to 20 cc/min. A phaco chop technique with a Beckert instrument or a 1.75 mm Nagahara chopping instrument is used to remove the two halves. The residual peripheral cortex is removed with the irritation/aspiration handpiece.

The chamber and bag are re-inflated with viscoelastics. A Crozafon punch is then used to remove 1.0 to 1.5 mm of trabecular meshwork, although the sclerostomy can be performed with a diamond knife (Fig. 10–5). The intraocular lens is then folded and placed into the capsular bag (Fig. 10–6). For many years, a silicone lens was the only foldable lens available,

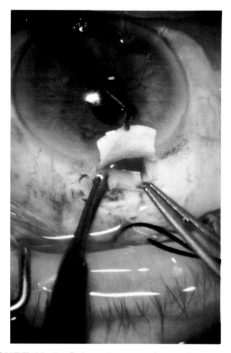

FIGURE 10–5. Sclerostomy performed.

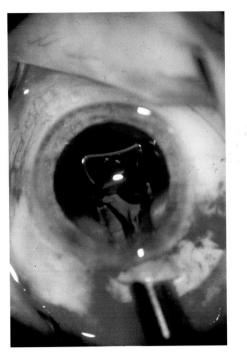

FIGURE 10–6. Insertion of a plate haptic silicone intraocular lens.

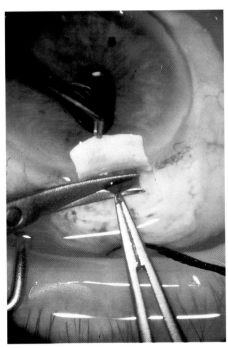

FIGURE 10–7. Peripheral iridectomy performed.

and both single (Chiron and Staar) and three piece lenses were used.[32] However, at this time I prefer a 6.0 mm acrylic lens. These tend to have fewer giant cell deposits on them and require fewer capsulotomies.

Acetylcholine (Miochol) is injected to produce miosis. A small peripheral iridectomy is performed (Fig. 10–7), although in large myopic eyes this may not be required. Some surgeons do not use an iridectomy at all, (Brad Shingleton, *personal communication*). The visco elastic is removed. The trabeculectomy flap is secured at the two corners with a 10-0 monofilament nylon suture.

The conjunctiva is re-apposed at the limbus with a 10-0 vicryl suture (Fig. 10–8), or a B-U 100 or VAS 10-4 needle (Ethicon) using a running horizontal mattress suture.[33] First, the suture is passed from cornea to conjunctiva and then tied. The needle is used to go conjunctiva to corneal surface and then cornea back to conjunctival surface. This is repeated every 0.5 mm until it is completed. It is tied onto itself and cut.

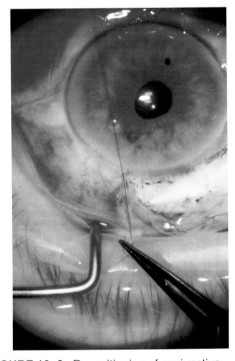

FIGURE 10–8. Repositioning of conjunctiva.

BSS on a syringe is then used to deepen the chamber and inflate the bleb. The wound is checked with fluorescein for water tightness.

A collagen shield soaked in Decadron^R and Ancef^R is placed on the eye. Usually no patch is applied.

▪ Postoperative Management

Patients are usually treated as a trabeculectomy. *Cycloplegia is used, frequent topical steroids, and antibiotics.* Once the chamber is stable, in 1 to 2 weeks, the cycloplegia and the antibiotic are stopped. Steroids may be used for 4 to 6 weeks.

Postoperative suture lysis may be used to modulate the pressure. If mitomycin has been used, suture lysis may be effective up to 3 to 4 weeks following surgery. If one does not have access to an Argon laser, releasable sutures can be used.

▪ Complications

Among the complications experienced with this combination procedure are hyphema, PCO, choroidal detachment, wound leaks, hypotonous maculopathy, misdirection syndrome, encapsulated bleb, and IOL shifting. There are certainly different complications of the combined procedure when compared with either cataract extraction or trabeculectomy alone. There are also complications related to the use of antimetabolites.

Hyphema is seen quite frequently, particularly if a peripheral iridectomy is done. These usually are self-limited and do not require intervention. They may be visually significant, but again are self-limited.

Choroidal detachments occur particularly in patients that have been on aqueous suppressants and those that start with a high intraocular pressure, often without any predisposition. If there is no wound leak, most choroidals are self-limited. Intervention is not needed unless they become "kissing choroidals." Treatment includes increasing cycloplegia, steroids, and occasionally deepening with viscoelastic agents.

Drainage with viscoelastic chamber deepening is rarely needed. I have seen peripheral choroidals last weeks before reabsorbing, and urge patience in their management.

Wound leaks occur approximately 5% of the time, especially when Mitomycin was used. These cases may be difficult to treat. If the leak is small, a large disposable contact lens may allow the leak to seal. If the leak is large or does not respond to the contact lens, I will place a 10-0 Vicryl suture in on a BV100 Ethicon needle, this can be done at the slit lamp with topical anesthesia. This will suffice for most leaks. Cyanoacrylic glue may be used if the leak is small. The area needs to be dried temporarily with a Weck-cel sponge and a drop of glue is placed. I usually cover it with a contact lens for comfort.

A more serious complication is hypotonous maculopathy (Fig. 10–9). The most susceptible group appear to be the young, female, myope who receive Mitomycin C (mmc). In this group I avoid using Mitomycin C. In fact, in any patient where mmc is used, make sure the eye is not soft at the end of the surgery and that the eye holds fluid. If hypotonous maculopathy occurs, there is usually two to three lines of vision lost, even if the pressure is brought up quickly by re-suturing the flap. Prevention is of paramount importance.

With encapsulated blebs, a 5FU injection of 10 mg into the bleb with lysis of the bleb may

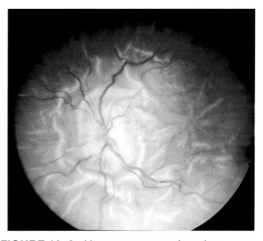

FIGURE 10–9. Hypotonous maculopathy.

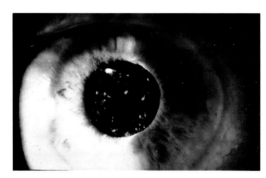

FIGURE 10–10. A Nd-YAG laser may be used to break the hyaloid face.

reduce the pressure in about 50% of the cases. Addition of anti-glaucoma medications may be required to reduce the pressure to a safe level.

Misdirection syndrome (malignant glaucoma) can be seen following combined procedures. Usually the eye has a shallow chamber, no leak, a peripheral iridectomy, and a high pressure. Many of these will respond to cycloplegia (atropine 1% tid or qid). Occasionally, a Nd-YAG laser may be used to break the hyaloid face and redirect the fluid anteriorly (Fig. 10–10). However, in stubborn cases, the most definitive way to attack misdirection syndrome is with pars plana vitrectomy. If the chamber shallows occasionally, the IOL may shift anteriorly. If the pupil shifts behind the implant, this may require re-deepening with viscoelastic.

■ Tips and Pearls

1. Good exposure is important and if there is a large brow, I would suggest doing cataract surgery through a temporal clear cornea incision. Place a single suture and then move superiorly for the trabeculectomy. If you plan to use mmc, you must not get any of it into the eye, I would use the mmc before removing the cataract by preparing the superior site and then rotate temporarily for the cataract surgery. Since hypotony is a possibility, I would suggest using a suture for the corneal wound. It can be removed within one or two weeks.

2. A tenonectomy is usually not performed unless there is likely to be trouble using a suture lysis procedure postoperatively. There may actually be an increased incidence of encapsulated blebs in patients that have had a tenonectomy.

3. Many patients that have been on miotics will have adhesions from the iris to the lens. It is necessary to break these and I usually remove any fibrotic membranes on the capsule prior to attempting a capsulorhexis.

4. Hydrodissection is quite important, especially in cases of pseudoexfoliation. The zonules and capsule are weak and rotations need to be very elegant. Cortical removal is difficult in patients with pseudoexfoliation and in this group one needs to use care to reduce zonular stress by removing small amounts of cortex and using side to side maneuvers rather than pulling directly from the capsule.

5. I use large lenses to reduce the chance of the IOL shifting. Plate lenses placed in the bag cannot have a pupillary capture, but there tends to be a higher incidence of giant cell deposits on them, and you must be careful to do a small YAG laser capsulotomy to reduce chances of a posterior migration of the lens.

REFERENCES

1. Krupin T, Feitl ME, Bishop KL. Postoperative intraocular pressure rise in open-angle glaucoma patients after cataract of combined cataract-filtration surgery. Ophthalmol 1989;96:579–584.
1. Mamalis N, Lohner S, Rand AN, et al. Combined phacoemulsification, intraocular lens implantation, and trabeculectomy. J Cataract Refract Surg 1996;22:467–473.
2. Gayton JL, Ledford JK. Combined phacoemulsification and trabeculectomy. Ann Ophthalmol 1995;27:27–32.
3. Metz D, Ackerman S, Lish AJ, et al. Phacotrabeculectomy with posterior chamber lens insertion in early glaucoma. Ann Ophthalmol 1995;27:231–235.
4. Shingleton BJ, Jacobson LM, Kuperwaser MC. Comparison of combined cataract and glaucoma surgery using planned extracapsular and phacoemulsification techniques. Ophthalmic Surg Laser 1995;26:414–419.
5. Steward WC, Sine CS, Carlson AN. Three-millimeter versus 6-mm incisions in combined phacoemulsifica-

tion and trabeculectomy. Ophthalmic Surg Laser 1996;27:832–838.
6. Cohen JS, Greff LJ, Novack GD, et al. A placebo-controlled double-masked evaluation of mitomycin c in combined glaucoma and cataract procedures. Ophthalmol 1996;103:1934–1942.
7. Lederer CM. Combined cataract extraction with intraocular lens implant and mitomycin-augmented trabeculectomy. Ophthalmol 1996;103:1025–1034.
8. Ruderman JM, Fundingsland B, Meyer MA. Combined phacoemulsification and trabeculectomy with mitomycin c. J Cataract Refract Surg 1996; 22:1085–1090.
9. Munden PM, Alward WLM. Combined phacoemulsification, posterior chamber intraocular lens implantation, and trabeculectomy with mitomycin c. Am J Ophthalmol 1995;119:20–29.
10. Gayton JL, Van Der Karr MA, Sanders V. Combined cataract and glaucoma procedures using temporal cataract surgery. J Cataract Refract Surg 1996;22:1485–1491.
11. Gous PNJ, Roux P. Preliminary report of sutureless phacotrabeculectomy through a modified self-sealing scleral tunnel incision. J Cataract Refract Surg 1995; 21:160–169.
12. Arnold PN. No-stitch phacotrabeculectomy. J Cataract Refract Surg 1996;22:253–260.
13. Bloomberg LB. Modified trabeculectomy/trabeculotomy with no-stitch cataract surgery. J Cataract Refract Surg 1996;22:14–22.
14. Hurvitz LM. 5-FU supplemented phacoemulsification, posterior chamber intraocular lens implantation, and trabeculectomy. Ophthalmic Surg 1993;24:674–680.
14. Naveh N, Kottas R, Glovinsky, et al. The long-term effect on intraocular pressure of a procedure combining trabeculectomy and cataract surgery, as compared with trabeculectomy alone. Ophthalmic Surg 1990; 21:339–345.
15. Yu CBO, Chong NHV, Caesar RH, et al. Long-term results of combined cataract and glaucoma surgery versus trabeculectomy along in low-risk patients. J Cataract Refract Surg 1996;22:352–357.
16. Menezo JL, Maldonado MJ, Muñoz G, et al. Combined procedure for glaucoma and cataract: a retrospective study. J Cataract Refract Surg 1994;20:498–503.
17. Wedrich A, Menapace R, Radax U, et al. Long-term results of combined trabeculectomy and small incision cataract surgery. J Cataract Refract Surg 1995; 21:49–54.
18. Wishart PK, Austin MW. Combined cataract extraction and trabeculectomy: phacoemulsification compared with extracapsular technique. Ophthalmic Surg 1993;24:814–821.
19. Stewart WC, Crinkley CMC, Carlson AN. Results of trabeculectomy combined with phacoemulsification versus trabeculectomy combined with extracapsular cataract extraction in patients with advanced glaucoma. Ophthalmic Surg 1994;25:621–627.
20. Lyle WA, Jin JC. Comparison of 3- and 6-mm incision in combined phacoemulsification and trabeculectomy. Am J Ophthalmol 1991;111:189–196.
21. Park JH, Wertzman M, Caprioti J. Temporal corneal phacoemulsification combined with superior trabeculectomy. Arch Ophthalmol 1997;115:318–323.
22. O'Grady JM, Juzych MS, Shin DH, et al. Trabeculectomy, phacoemulsification and posterior chamber lens implantation with an without 5FU. Am J Opthalmol 1993;116:594–599.
23. Wong PC, Ruderman JM, Krupin T, et al. 5-Flourouracil after primary combined filtration surgery. Am J Ophthalmol 1994;117:149–154.
24. Shin DH, Simone PA, Song MS, et al. Adjunctive subconjunctival mitomycin c in glaucoma triple procedure. Ophthalmol 1995;102:1550–1558.
25. Shin DH, Hughes BA, Song MS, et al. Primary glaucoma triple procedure with or without adjunctive mitomycin: prognostic factors for filtration failure. Ophthalmol 1996;103:1925–1933.
26. Berefsha JS, Brown SVC. Limbus versus fornix based conjunctival flaps in combined phacoemulsification and mitomycin c trabeculectomy surgery. Ophthalmol 1997;104:187–196.
27. Masket S. Preplaced inferior iris suture method for small pupil phacoemulsification. J Cataract Refract Surg 1992;18:318–322.
28. Mackool RJ. Small pupil enlargement during cataract extraction. J Cataract Refract Surg 1991;18:523–526.
29. Joseph J, Wang HS. Phacoemulsification with poorly dilated pupils. J Cataract Refract Surg 1993;18:551–556.
30. Fine IH. Pupiloplasty for small pupil phacoemulsification. J Cataract Refract Surg 1994;20:192–196.
31. Densmore SC. Modified stretch technique for small pupil phacoemulsification with topical anesthesia. J Cataract Refract Surg 1996;22:27–30.
32. Gandolfi SA, Vecchi M. 5-Flourouracil in combined trabeculectomy and clear-cornea phacoemulsification with posterior chamber intraocular lens implantation. Ophthalmol 1997;104:181–186.
32. Kosman A, Wishart PK, Ridges PJG. Silicone versus poly methyl methacrylate lenses in combined phacoemulsification and trabeculectomy. J Cataract Refract Surg 1997;23:97–105.
33. Liss RP, Scholes GN, Crandall AS. Glaucoma filtration surgery: new horizontal mattress closure of conjunctival incision. Ophthal Surg 1991; 22:298–300.

11

Phacoemulsification in Pseudoexfoliation

I. HOWARD FINE AND RICHARD S. HOFFMAN

Phacoemulsification in the presence of pseudoexfoliation of the lens presents surgeons with particular challenges. Intraoperative and postoperative complications such as zonular dialysis, capsule tears, vitreous loss, and IOL decentration may be avoided with careful attention to detail and elegant surgical technique. Improvements in phacoemulsification technology, intraocular lenses, and new capsular supporting rings offer surgeons the capability of performing safer surgery in these patients. Herein we present many of the challenges and options for managing cataract extraction in the presence of pseudoexfoliation.

Cataract surgery in the presence of pseudoexfoliation of the lens presents surgeons with unusual challenges. In addition to a higher incidence of glaucoma, these patients have loss of zonular integrity occasionally associated with lens subluxation and pupils that dilated poorly. Although the use of phacoemulsification in experienced hands has resulted in a low incidence of intraoperative and postoperative complications such as zonular dialysis, capsule tears, vitreous loss, and IOL decentration,[1] special care should still be exercised when performing cataract surgery in these patients. Improvements in phacoemulsification technology, technique, and new capsular supporting rings will ultimately enable these patients to undergo cataract surgery with even fewer complications.

■ Technique

Glaucoma

Poorly controlled glaucoma with concomitant cataract and pseudoexfoliation is best managed by a glaucoma triple procedure. We prefer the utilization of a limbal conjunctival incision without vertical releasing incisions and a self sealing scleral tunnel incision (without vertical releasing incisions) located superiorly through which phacoemulsification is performed. A Crozafon-De Laage Punch (Moria #18069) is used to disrupt the posterior corneal lip, creating a fistula which usually results in a diffuse shallow bleb that filters posteriorly. The conjunctival incision is sutured to the limbus at the conclusion of the procedure. Although this is our preferred method, any combined technique can be used with or without the use of antimetabolites.

For patients with glaucoma who do not need filtration surgery at the time of cataract surgery, we prefer our usual clear corneal incision form the temporal periphery. This allows the entire procedure to take place through avascular tissue and does not prejudice future filtration surgery in a superior location.

Small Pupils

The small pupil can be managed in a variety of ways including sector iridectomy, iris hooks, iris rings, and pupillary stretching with or without the use of multiple half-width sphincterotomies.[2] At present, we find the Beehler Pupil Dilator (Moria #19009) to be uniformly applicable in the presence of small pupils. It usually stretches the pupil to 6 to 7 mm while creating tiny microsphincterotmies circumferentially around the pupil (Fig. 11–1A to C). The pupil can then be mechanically reduced at the end of the procedure with a Lester hook supplemented with an intraocular miotic. Pupils enlarged in this manner maintain a good cosmetic appearance and an ability to react to light but may require miotic drops for some time following cataract surgery to avoid synechiae to the capsulorhexis margin.

Capsulorhexis

Weak zonules present particularly challenging situations during phacoemulsification. Of utmost importance is to not challenge the integrity of the zonules by over-pressurizing the eye. This can occur following peri- or retrobulbar injection with digital or Honan pressure, overexpanding the anterior chamber with viscoelastic prior to capsulotomy, or utilizing an excessively high bottle height during phacoemulsification.

Due to the lack of zonular integrity, frequently it is difficult to actually perforate the capsule to begin a capsulorhexis. We use pinch-type forceps such as the Kershner Capsulorhexis cystotome forceps (Rhein Medical 05–2320) or the Rhein Capsulorhexis Cystotome Forceps (Rhein Medical 05–2326) which allow one to grasp the capsule to start the tear rather than beginning the capsulotomy with a perforation by downward pressure on the lens. This is especially important in fibrosed capsules which cannot be perforated by a needle. When one purchases the capsule with a pinch and tears it, the tear will commence at

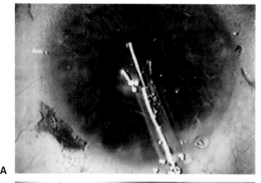

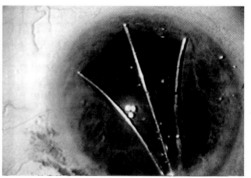

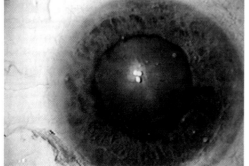

FIGURE 11–1. (A) Small pupil with Beehler pupil dilator inserted through temporal clear corneal incision. **(B)** Temporal iris is engaged with mounted hook on undersurface of instrument and retracted while the dilator is opened to stretch the pupil at four points 360 degrees. **(C)** Appearance of the pupil following mechanical dilation.

the edge of the fibrosis, usually at the pupillary margin.

During the capsulotomy, special care and attention are required, because traction on the capsule can unzip weakened zonules. If there are areas of missing zonules, centripetal traction on the capsular flap may result in further damage to the adjacent weakened zonules. Techniques of two-handed capsulotomy using tangential forces as described by Neuhann[3] are excellent adjunctive techniques in situations with loose zonules. After the capsulotomy has been started, the capsular flap is stabilized with the forceps through the main incision, while a second instrument such as a bifurcated spatula is introduced through the side-port incision. Slight backward traction is placed on the flap with the forceps with the second instrument directly advances the torn edge in a tangential manner.

Capsulorhexis size is extremely important in patients with pseudoexfoliation. Ideal capsulorhexis size is felt to be 5.5 to 6.0 mm or larger in routine patients.[4] We believe it should be at least 6.0 mm in pseudoexfoliaton cases, since a larger capsulorhexis leaves a smaller burden of lens epithelial cells postoperatively than smaller capsulorhexis. Residual lens epithelial cells participate in metaplasia and extracellular matrix deposition, ultimately resulting in capsular fibrosis.[5] Patients with pseudoexfoliation are particularly susceptible to marked shrinkage of the rhexis, because the strong forces of fibrosis and contraction are unopposed by strong zonular traction.[6] Thus, a larger capsulorhexis should decrease the incidence of symptomatic capsule contraction by decreasing the number of epithelial cells able to participate in the fibrosis process and allow for a larger final rhexis diameter once capsule contraction has ultimately ceased to progress.

Hydrodissection and Hydrodelineation

Cortical cleaving hydrodissection[7] requires extremely careful maneuvers especially when one decompresses the bag after having performed the posterior fluid wave. It is important to do this very gently and to utilize multiple locations for partial cortical cleaving hydrodissection injections with gentle central lens decompression. This should alleviate the chances of depressing the lens with excessive forces which would tear zonules.

Hydrodelineation is a useful technique in pseudoexfoliation, since it produces an epinuclear shell as an important added safeguard. During both hydrodissection and hydrodelineation, it is wise to keep the cannula in a position slightly depressing the posterior lip of the incision. This will ensure easy egress out of the eye for either viscoelastic or fluid should one overinflate the spaces with balanced salt solution.

Phacoemulsification

One must use extreme caution during manipulation of the lens so as to not tear zonules. Two-handed rotations of the lens nucleus are wise, since the forces can be truly tangential and can be divided by utilizing opposite sides of the same meridian. Grooving also requires special care, since there is a tendency to put posterior pressure on the nucleus. High cavitation tips, such as the Kelman tip on the Alcon System 20,000 Legacy, are a great advantage, since they can obliterate nuclear material in advance of the tip without exerting forces on the lens or the lens zonules. The particular configuration of the Kelman tip allows for a variation of the Gimbel "phaco sweep" procedure[8] where the initial groove can be formed, and then, without rotating the lens, a lateral and rotational motion of the phaco probe grooves in a lateral direction (Fig. 11-2).

One may also help stabilize the nucleus during grooving. We find it best not to perform downslope sculpting, because nudging the nucleus in the direction in which one is sculpting can put unnecessary traction on the zonules in the subincisional area. If the nucleus is going to be stabilized at all, it can be stabilized through the side port with a second instrument. In addition to stabilization, one can actually push the nucleus toward the phaco tip to maximize the efficiency of the tip, and at the same time, elevate the lens slightly.

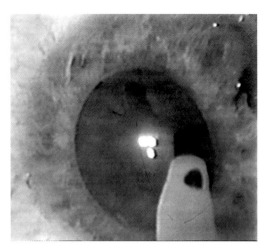

FIGURE 11–2. Following formation of a vertical groove in the meridian of the incision, a groove perpendicular to the first is formed without rotating the lens by moving the phaco probe laterally and with a rotational movement.

For lens cracking, we recommend nonrotational cracking as described by Fine, Maloney, and Dillman.[9] This appears to be the least traumatic method for cracking the nucleus and dismantling it into quadrants that are easy to mobilize. The epinuclear shell helps stabilize the nucleus and is useful during the mobilization of the four quadrants because all of the phaco and mechanical forces can be confined within the epinuclear space reducing stress on the zonules, as well as the capsule.

Cortical aspiration represents the biggest threat to the zonules during phacoemulsification of cataracts in pseudoexfoliation patients, because the greatest amount of traction can be placed on the zonules during this step of the procedure. Prior use of cortical cleaving hydrodissection is important in reducing traction on zonules and facilitating removal of most if not all of the cortex during flipping and evaluation of the epinuclear shell. We recommend cortical cleanup not be performed in these cases until after implantation of the IOL. In the presence of pseudoexfoliation, we usually utilize a foldable lens with PMMA haptics sized for bag placement. Aspiration of residual cortex is safer after the lens has been implanted due to stabilization of the capsular bag by the implant.

We also recommend tangential traction on the cortex with the I/A tip rather than stripping centrally in order to maximize forces on a few cortical/capsular connections at a time (Fig. 11–3). If there are areas of zonular dehiscence, it is important to strip tangentially toward the dehiscence rather than away from it since stripping away from the area of dehiscence would localize forces on weakened zonules which might lead to unzipping of the zonular dehiscence.

Capsular Ring

The newest and most important adjunctive therapy in addressing cataracts with pseudoexfoliation has been the use of a capsular ring (Morcher Type 14 and Type 14A) as described by Witschel and Legler.[10] The endocapsular ring is a polymethylmethacrylate ring with expanded ends which contain positioning holes. The ring comes in two sizes: 10 mm (Type 14) for routine cases and 12 mm (Type 14A) for high myopes.

When placed within the capsular bag, which is approximately 10 mm in diameter, the ring keeps the bag on stretch and provides several advantages. It prevents concentration of forces on individual zonules by distributing all forces applied to any point on the capsulorhexis to

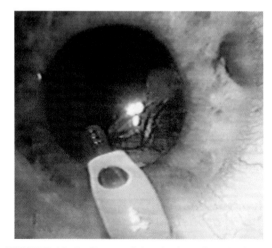

FIGURE 11–3. Tangential stripping of cortical material rather than centripetal stripping maximizes forces on a few cortical/capsular connections at a time.

the entire zonular apparatus. It also keeps the bag on stretch throughout the procedure, allowing for greater safety during all intraocular manipulations. Finally, the continuous pressure of the ring against the capsular fornices acts to bolster any residual zonular traction on the capsule and counter the force of constriction following metaplasia and fibrosis of the capsulorhexis.

We have found it best to place the ring in the bag immediately after the capsulorhexis is completed. The ring is slipped into the incision and fed under the rhexis with a forceps while the second hand guides it with a Lester hook through the side port incision (Figs. 11-4A to D). Once the ring is in place, cortical cleaving hydrodissection is performed followed by hydrodelineation, and then, the remainder of the procedure can be done utilizing many of the guidelines listed above. Although cortical cleaving hydrodissection may have been performed, the endocapsular ring holds much of the cortex pressed up against the capsular fornices requiring an additional amount of force to remove the cortex with the irrigation/aspiration handpiece. Despite this, there is a great deal more safety during the procedure because of the equal distribution of forces by the ring and stabilization of the capsular bag.

The safety of a plate haptic lens in the presence of an endocapsular ring is in question due to the outward force of the ring. The ring may allow for decentration of the plate haptic IOL because it continues to keep the bag in a highly expanded state. In addition, YAG laser

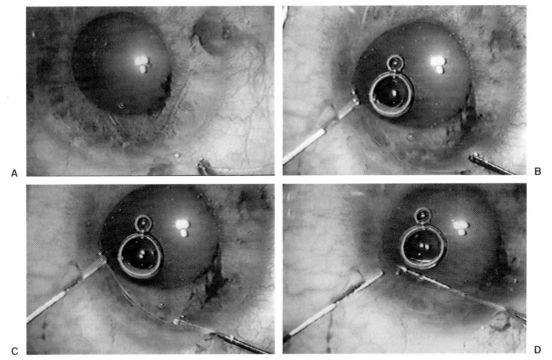

FIGURE 11-4. Capsular ring insertion. **(A)** Following capsulorhexis and prior to cortical cleaving hydrodissection, the capsular ring is inserted through the clear corneal incision with a forceps. The leading eyelet is placed under the capsulorhexis into the capsular fornix. **(B)** Once the ring is inserted to the point that the trailing eyelet has reached the incision, a Lester hook is placed in the trailing eyelet while a second Lester hook is placed through the paracentesis. **(C)** The right-handed Lester hook then inserts the ring further as it enters the anterior chamber while the second instrument helps guide the capsular ring. **(D)** As the trailing eyelet reaches the edge of the capsulorhexis, the right-handed Lester hook is rotated clockwise 90 degrees in order to disengage the eyelet from the hook. The inherent tension of the ring will place the trailing end in the capsular fornix.

capsulotomy, which may be followed by tears of the posterior capsule out to the equator, could allow a plate haptic lens to drop into the vitreous cavity since older style lenses are not fixated by the capsule.[11] It is possible that the newer designed plate haptic lenses with fenestrations or half-haptics will be safer in the presence of an endocapsular ring since they have been shown to fixate to the capsular bag.[12,13]

■ Tips and Pearls

1. Patients with pseudoexfoliation of the lens have weakened zonules. Do not challenge the integrity of the zonules by overpressurizing the eye.
2. Capsulorhexis size is extremely important in patients with pseudoexfoliation and should be at least 6.0 mm.
3. Cortical cleanup should not be performed in these cases until after the implantation of the IOL. Aspiration of the residual cortex is safer after the lens has been implanted due to stabilization of the capsular bag by the implant.
4. In the presence of pseudoexfoliation, the intraocular lens should have PMMA haptics to increase haptic resistance and attempt to prevent capsule contraction and lens decentration.
5. We recommend tangential traction on the cortex with the I/A tip rather than stripping centrally in order to maximize forces on a few cortical/capsular connections at a time. If there are areas of zonular dehiscence, it is important to strip tangentially toward the dehiscence rather than away from it since stripping away from the area of dehiscence would localize forces on weakened zonules.
6. Placing an endocapsular ring prior to phacoemulsification keeps the lens capsule taut preventing concentration of forces on individual zonules by distributing all forces applied to any point on the capsulorhexis to the entire zonular apparatus. This results in greater safety during all intraocular manipulations.

■ Conclusion

Phacoemulsification in the presence of pseudoexfoliation presents surgeons with the possibility of many complications which are less likely to occur in the absence of pseudoexfoliation. Specialized techniques are available which should allow the surgeon to both avoid and cope with the various intraoperative difficulties which may become manifest during cataract surgery in these patients. One of the newest devices available to assist in managing these cases is the endocapsular ring. It offers the potential benefits of fewer intra and postoperative complications by means of capsular stabilization. Future studies will ultimately determine all of the benefits and indications of the endocapsular ring.

REFERENCES

1. Osher RH, Cioni RJ, Gimbel HV, Crandall AS. Cataract surgery in patients with pseudoexfoliation syndrome. Eur J Implant Ref Surg 1993; 5:46–50.
2. Fine IH. Phacoemulsification in the presence of small pupil. In: Steinert RF (ed). Cataract Surgery: Technique, Complications, and Management. Philadelphia: WB Saunders; 1995;199–208.
3. Neuhann TF. Capsulorhexis. In: Steinert RF (ed). Cataract Surgery: Technique, Complications, and Management. Philadelphia: WB Saunders; 1995;134–142.
4. Joo CK, Shin JA, Kim JH. Capsular opening contraction after continuous curvilinear capsulorhexis and intraocular lens implantation. J Cataract Refract Surg 1996; 22:585–590.
5. Ishibashi T, Araki H, Sugai S, et al. Anterior capsular opacification in monkey eyes with posterior chamber intraocular lenses. Arch Ophthalmol 1993; 111:1685–1690.
6. Davison JA. Capsule contraction syndrome. J Cataract Refract Surg 1993; 19:582–589.
7. Fine IH. Cortical cleaving hydrodissection. J Cataract Refract Surg 1992; 18:508–512.
8. Gimbel HV, Chin PK. Phaco sweep. J Cataract Refract Surg 1995; 21:493–503.
9. Fine IH, Maloney WF, Dillman DM. Crack and flip phacoemulsification technique. Cataract Refract Surg 1993; 19:797–802.
10. Witchel BM, Legler U. New aproaches to zonular cases: the capsular ring. Audiovisual J Cataract Implant Surg 1993; 9 (4).

11. Levy JH, Pisacano AM, Anello RD. Displacement of bag placed hydrogel lenses into the vitreous following neodynium: YAG laser capsulotomy. J Cataract Refract Surg 1990; 16:563–566.
12. Apple DJ. Enhancement of silicone plate IOL fixation by the use of positioning holes in the lens haptic. American Society of Cataract and Refractive Surgery Symposium, Seattle, WA, June 1996.
13. Mamalis N. Comparison of silicon plate haptic IOL models AA-4203 and AA-4203F in a rabbit model. American Society of Cataract and Refractive Surgery Symposium, Seattle, WA, June 1996.

12

Phacoemulsification in Subluxated Cataracts

ANDRES CORÉT, JORGE VILLAR-KURI,
YOSHIHIRO TOKUDA, AND LUIS W. LU

The surgical management of the cataract associated with zonular dialysis is a real challenge for the ophthalmic surgeon. Due to recent advances in equipment and instrumentation, better surgical techniques and understanding of fluidics, the surgeon will be able to perform relative safe cataract surgery in presence of compromised zonules.

In presence of mild loss of zonular fibers, cataract surgery can be managed by conventional phacoemulsification and implantation techniques, while extremely loose cataracts may require an intracapsular method.[1] When more than 4 or 5 clock hours of capsular zonular support are missing, many surgeons prefer performing an intracapsular cataract extraction with implantation of an anterior chamber or sutured posterior chamber intraocular lens (IOL). Traditionally, congenital or acquired zonulocapsular pathology has not allowed implantation of a posterior chamber IOL in the capsular bag nor in the ciliary sulcus. For this reason, new techniques have been designed to correct the deficiencies of the natural support for the IOL, as with the use of endocapsular rings to expand the equatorial portion of the capsule, or artificially modifying this anatomical support by suturing the anterior capsule to the sclera. IOL in-the-bag suture is a new approach to zonular dehiscence.[2]

■ The Capsular Ring

Description

The capsular ring is made of one-piece PMMA CQ UV C-F-M and is available in different sizes depending of their use in patients with emmetropia, low, or high myopia. The 10 mm capsular ring is the easiest to implant and the most commonly used. Capsular rings of 11 and 12 mm in diameter are reserved for myopic and high myopic patients. At present, they are mainly distributed by two companies, Morcher[3] and Corneal Paris.[4]

We have available the technical data from Morcher. The rings were designed in cooperation with Dr. Witschel Morcher. The Type 14 is for normal axial length eyes, while types 14A and 14C are for myopic eyes. Type 14:12.3–10 mm; Type 14A:14.5–12 mm; and Type 14C: 13.0–11 mm.

The higher figures represent the diameter of the ring as it lies in the packaged container, while the lower figures represent the diameter at which the ring is totally round, i.e., in the capsular bag.

The Type 14 has an haptic thickness of 0.15 mm and is used for the circular expansion of the capsular bag and the prevention of capsular fibrosis in eyes with average axial length and has been available since 1991. The Type 14A (1992 design) has a 0.20 mm of haptic thickness and this was designed particularly rigid because of the high tendency of capsular shrinkage in highly myopic eyes with 28.0 mm or more of axial length. It has been recommended implantation of ring 14A in combination with a security suture to facilitate its implantation. The capsular tension ring Type 14C was developed in 1994 for its implantation in myopic eyes. As compared with Type 14A, Type 14C has a diameter of 11.0 mm with a thinner design at the ends of the ring. The haptic thickness is then 0.15/0.20 mm, to facilitate its implantation. Long-term studies have shown a properly expanded bag in myopic eyes. The Type 14C is recommended for eyes with under 17D.

Implantation Technique

After filling the capsular bag with viscoelastic material, the ring is introduced through the cataract incision with the convexity to the left or to the side in which the paracentesis was made to allow easier manipulation (Fig. 12–1). Once the ring is being introduced in the bag, a

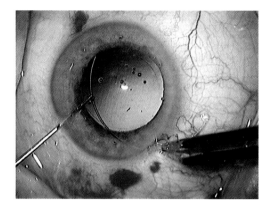

FIGURE 12—2. Guiding the ring into the bag.

buttonhole spatula is placed through the paracentesis guiding the ring and preventing the continuous circular capsulotomy (CCC) from getting deformed (Fig. 12–2). To complete implantation of the ring, it may be helpful to use a similar spatula, introduced through the phacoemulsification incision (Fig. 12–3). This step is certainly more complicated and depends on the size and rigidity of the ring to be implanted.

Indications

To Prevent Capsular Contraction with Resulting IOL Dislocation

The most common indication in this group is pseudoexfoliation of the lens capsule which is associated with poor pupillary dilation, weak zonular support, and a high incidence of cap-

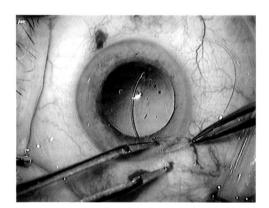

FIGURE 12–1. Initial stage of the endocapsular ring insertion.

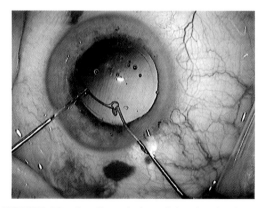

FIGURE 12—3. Completion of the ring implantation.

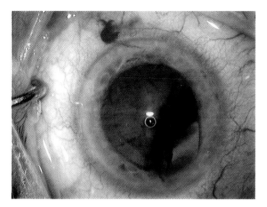

FIGURE 12—4. Vitreous prolapse.

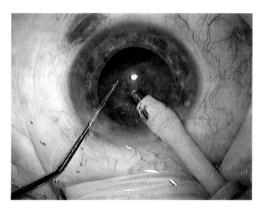

FIGURE 12—6. Zonular disinsertion during phacoemulsification.

sular bag contraction with IOL decentration, especially in cases where foldable lenses and flexible haptics have been implanted. In patients with very weak zonules, the implantation of a capsular ring and an IOL with PMMA haptics will be indicated.[5]

Intraoperative Partial Zonular Disinsertion

In this situation the ring is implanted at the time the zonular dehiscence is noticed, and no further phacoemulsification or cortex aspiration is performed until inserting the endocapsular ring. This prevents vitreous prolapse and wound incarceration (Fig. 12–4). An early sign of zonular weakness is the presence of radial folds in the anterior capsule at the time the CCC is started (Fig. 12–5). In this situation, a safe CCC will be difficult. The surgeon should be careful during nucleus rotation preventing zonular tension. If during phacoemulsification a zonular disinsertion with vitreous prolapse to the anterior chamber occurs (Fig. 12–6), stop the procedure, reform the capsular bag with viscoelastic material, and implant the endocapsular ring (Fig. 12–7). The surgeon should be able to complete the planned procedure without major complications (Fig. 12–8).

Obtain Pseudophakia in Subluxated Lenses

In these cases the degree of subluxation must be evaluated in a supine position (Fig. 12–9). The presence and density of a cataract, iridodonesis, phacodonesis, and the opposite eye must be determined.

A subluxated lens can induce optical aberrations difficult to correct with the use of con-

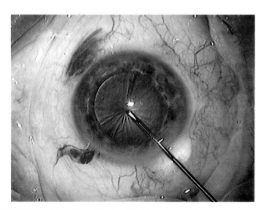

FIGURE 12—5. Radial folds at the time of capsulotomy as an early sign of zonular weakness.

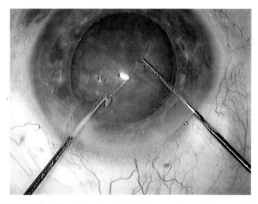

FIGURE 12—7. Implantation of endocapsular ring.

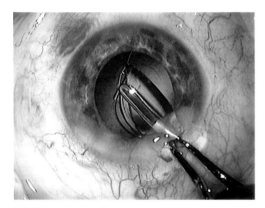

FIGURE 12—8. Completion of the planned procedure.

tact lenses or glasses. The astigmatism is induced by the equator of the lens, the motion of this subluxated lens, or the lens shape irregularity as a result of the partial loss of the zonular fibers. The high myopia that is usually associated, can be caused by the high refractive power of the peripheral zone of the lens or by the increase of its curvature due to the absence of zonular fibers. This optical alteration can cause monocular or binocular diplopia, anisometropia, or amblyopia in children. In cases of secondary visual disturbance in which vision cannot be corrected, surgery must be considered.

The classic approach has been a planned limbal or pars plana lensectomy, especially in cases of Marfan Syndrome. The use of the endocapsular ring would maintain the capsular bag and an IOL may then be inserted. The surgical technique is difficult, but if the intraocular compartments and pseudophakia are maintained, the risk of cystoid macular edema and retinal detachment frequently associated with Marfan Syndrome will be decreased.

The surgical technique is started with a small CCC where the anterior capsular folds can be observed. Hydrodissection and lens aspiration with the irrigation/aspiration cannula is performed. Flow rate, vacuum, and height of the infusion bottle are adjusted to prevent vitreous aspiration. It is important to use a low cohesive viscoelastic during the procedure. Once the lens is partially removed, the capsular ring is placed through the small CCC (Fig. 12–10). It is also feasible to insert the ring prior to the aspiration of the nucleus. Before the IOL insertion, the CCC must be enlarged so its edge will not be present at the pupillary area (Fig. 12–11). Insertion of a PMMA IOL with a 6.5 mm optical zone is preferred preventing having the edge of the IOL at the visual axis should it dislocate slightly. Scleral fixation of the capsular ring with sutures, may decrease the subluxation rate and prevent dislocation.

It is then important for the surgeon to be familiar with the use of the endocapsular ring and be able to use it correctly should a zonular dialysis be encountered. Attempted phacoemulsification or aspiration/irrigation without the ring will only increase the risk of surgical complications.

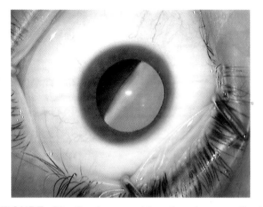

FIGURE 12—9. Lens subluxation in a patient with Marfan.

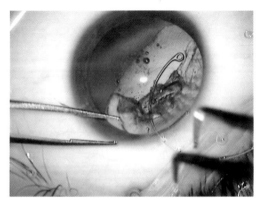

FIGURE 12—10. Introduction of a capsular ring after partial lens removal.

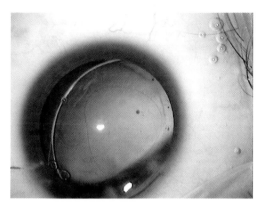

FIGURE 12—11. Enlarged capsulotomy.

■ Fixation of the Anterior Lens Capsule to the Sclera as a Support for a Posterior Chamber Intraocular Lens and as a Vitreous Container

Indications

This is indicated in patients with a 40 to 80% loss of the zonular fibers as a result of a congenital zonular pathology, that is, Marfan syndrome, or acquired as a result of previous trauma, in whom traditionally the implantation of a PC IOL is contraindicated.

Preoperative Evaluation

A careful preoperative evaluation should be performed with special attention to the zonular status, locating the area where the zonules are apparently intact. This has an important clinical value for the procedure since the incision must centered on that particular area. This will allow a safer approach to the anterior chamber and, manipulation of the surgical instruments without encountering vitreous. It is also important to observe the size and shape of the lens or subluxated cataract, presence of equatorial deformities, and the degree of dislocation. Pupillary dilation, integrity of the hyaloid and the location of the vitreous prolapse should also be evaluated.

IOL Selection

When selecting the IOL, considerations should be given to the IOL design. Foldable IOLs designed for in-the-bag implantation have known advantages. However, in most cases this type of IOL cannot be used since they are designed for capsular bag implantation with shorter overall length. They can be used in patients with a small anterior segment, in whom the lens will not dislocate even if they are sulcus fixated. These lenses have a large optical zone that will adequately cover the pupillary area. Unfortunately patients with Marfan Syndrome have a large anterior segment, and in these patients the IOL indicated is the one designed to be implanted in the ciliary sulcus. This type of IOL will decrease the risk of dislocation although these lenses require a larger incision.

Surgical Technique

The incision is made in the meridian where the zonules are considered to be intact. This procedure is considered difficult when the lens in subluxated nasally and superior (Fig. 12–12). The length of the incision depends on the type of IOL selected. If a foldable lens can be used, a 3 mm corneal incision is preferred. This incision should be enlarged to 3.8 to 4 mm to allow the IOL implantation. If this type of lens is not indicated, then the incision will be made at the limbus. The incision should be parallel to the limbus and enlarged to 7.5 mm in length to allow the insertion of the large optical zone intraocular lens.

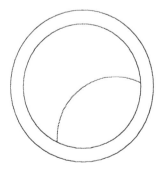

FIGURE 12—12. Surgeon's view of the left eye. Incision in the meridian where the zonules are considered to be intact.

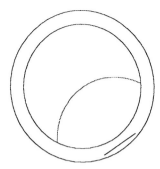

FIGURE 12—13. Schematic drawing of a clear corneal incision.

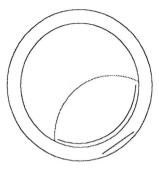

FIGURE 12—15. Tear extended with Vannas scissors.

The Incisions
If it is corneal (Fig. 12–13), the incision should be of 3 mm and single plane, preferably performed with a diamond blade. Otherwise an scleral tunnel incision is developed. Opposite to the cataract incision site, and after a conjunctival flap is developed, a scleral incision of 0.8 mm in length (and almost as deep) is performed at about 1.8 mm posterior to the limbus.

Capsulotomy
The anterior chamber is filled with high density viscoelastic material. A small capsular tear is constructed in the most peripheral area where the zonules are still intact (Fig. 12–14). With the Vannas scissors the tear is extended up to the level of the altered equator of the lens (Fig. 12–15).

Suturing the Capsule to the Sclera
Viscoelastic material is introduced beneath the anterior lens capsule and viscodisecction performed. A 10-0 Prolene suture preferably in a C-7 needle, is used to penetrate the flap of the anterior capsule as close to the capsular incision as possible (Figs. 12–16 and 12–17). A knot is tied outside the eye and is gently slid until it reaches the capsule. A square knot is eventually obtained (Fig. 12–18). These maneuvers must be gentle and precise to prevent a capsular tear. One end of the suture then is cut almost flush to the capsule.

Through the scleral incision opposite to the corneal or limbal cataract incision, a 25 gauge hypodermic needle is introduced with the bevel up (Fig. 12–19). The deepest scleral fibers are perforated, directing the tip initially towards the central part of the posterior chamber. The needle is then directed over the lens or subluxated cataract without touching it. Finally, the needle exits through the

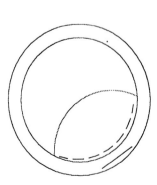

FIGURE 12—14. A small capsular tear performed.

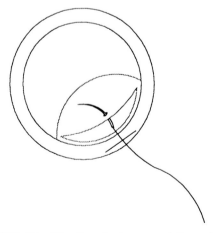

FIGURE 12—16. Needle is passed through the anterior capsular flap.

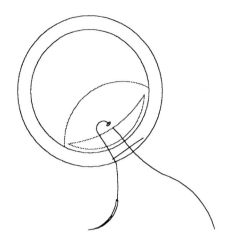

FIGURE 12—17. Needle is withdrawn.

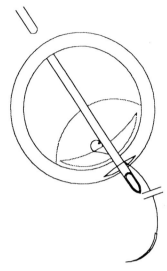

FIGURE 12—19. A 25 gauge needle is introduced bevel up.

corneal or limbal incision where the 10-0 nylon needle is inserted in the bore of the hypodermic needle, without changing its curvature (Fig. 12–20). The 10-0 nylon needle enters slightly tight which will prevent it to slide out when the hypodermic needle is pulled back (Fig. 12–21). This maneuver should spread out the anterior capsule with a slight tension (Figs. 12–22 and 12–23).

Phacoemulsification

The lens is then hydrodissected. The phaco tip is introduced while having the irrigation bottle at approximately 70% of the usual height. The anterior cortex and nucleus are aspirated with a vacuum of 30 mmHg and, short bursts of ultrasound power of 30 to 50% are used should the nucleus not be aspirated (Fig. 12–24). Caution should be taken to avoid capsular aspiration.

In few instances the ultrasound power might need to be raised for a harder nucleus. In these cases, nuclear fragmentation techniques that require nucleus expansion are not performed.

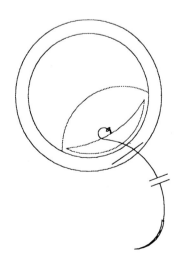

FIGURE 12—18. Square knot obtained.

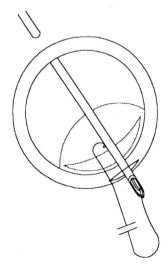

FIGURE 12—20. The needle of the 10-0 prolene suture is inserted in the bore.

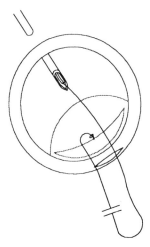

FIGURE 12—21. The 25 gauge needle is withdrawn.

Irrigation/Aspiration

Remaining cortical material is aspirated with the minimum vacuum possible for safe removal (Fig. 12–25). An angled tip is preferred for the subincisional area.

The anterior capsulotomy is enlarged under viscoelastic material (Fig. 12–26). The suture is now fixated to the sclera (Fig. 12–27).

IOL Insertion

The corneal or limbal incision is enlarged. Foldable lenses may be implanted while having the haptics tucked under the optical portion of

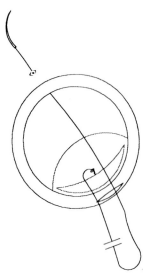

FIGURE 12—22. Ten-0 nylon suture exited through the scleral incision.

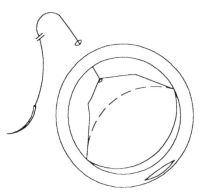

FIGURE 12—23. Spreading out the anterior capsule.

the folded IOL (Fig. 12–28). In the case of a rigid IOL, the haptic is placed directly in the sulcus at the level of the area of scleral-fixation. No rotation or pressure over the sutured capsule is applied. The proximal haptic is then implanted in the sulcus. Once the IOL is positioned, the excess of viscoelastic material is gently aspirated and the incision closed with 10-0 nylon suture (Fig. 12–29).

Small Subluxation

In those cases in which the subluxation is 4 to 5 clock hours, phacoemulsification can be performed through a corneal or limbal incision and away from the area of zonular dehiscence to prevent accidental aspiration of the vitreous. IOL in-the-bag implantation is performed placing the haptics in the meridian of the zonular disinsertion.

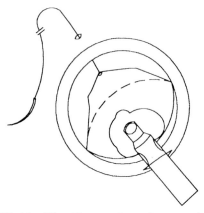

FIGURE 12—24. Slow-motion phacoemulsification.

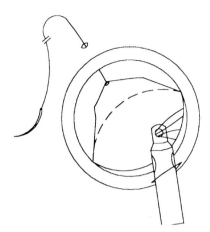

FIGURE 12—25. Removal of cortical material.

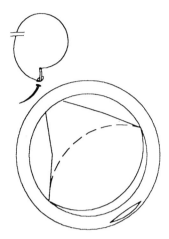

FIGURE 12—27. The 10-0 nylon suture is fixated to the sclera.

■ IOL In-The-Bag Suture for Zonular Dehiscence

The concept of in-the-bag IOL suture fixation is new, but the technique itself is simple and very similar to the conventional method. The difficulty of suture fixation is unaffected by the presence of the capsular bag, and an advantage is that the lens capsule is left intact.

The reason why in-the-bag IOL suture fixation has not been performed much in the past is not that the technique is difficult. Rather, the problem has been that extraction procedures for cataracts with lens subluxation or weak zonulae are difficult. Accordingly, the key to the success of this surgery lies in keeping the capsular bag as intact as possible prior to the process of IOL fixation.

In case of vitreous herniation into the anterior chamber, anterior vitrectomy is first performed. The phaco manipulations should be done gently and carefully so as not to extent the zonular dehiscence. Sufficient hydrodissection after the anterior capsulorhexis, completely separating the nucleus and epinucleus from the lens capsule, prevents stretching of the capsular bag by the aspiration flow.

During phaco and cortex aspiration, the capsular bag should be extended using a blunt hook inserted at the equator of the area of zonular dehiscence. In cases of greater than 120 degrees zonular dehiscence, it is difficult to extent the lens capsule with the hook alone, and a capsular tension ring must be used (Figs. 12–30 and 12–31). The implantation of

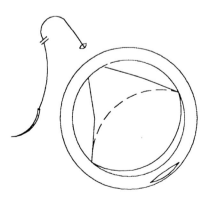

FIGURE 12—26. The anterior capsulotomy is enlarged.

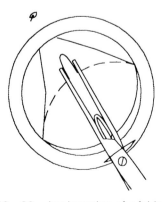

FIGURE 12—28. Implantation of a foldable lens.

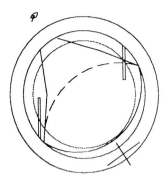

FIGURE 12—29. Wound closure with a single 10-0 nylon suture.

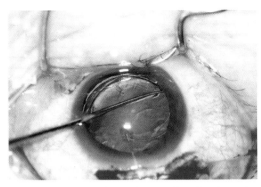

FIGURE 12—31. Capsular tension ring insertion.

the ring before phacoemulsification fully extends the capsular bag, preventing extension of the zonular dehiscence and vitreous herniation, thus permitting phaco and cortex aspiration to be performed safely.

Surgical Technique

The IOL haptics are sutured at the position of zonular dehiscence in order to extend the loose capsular bag. The suture penetration procedures are virtually the same as those of the conventional no-capsule suturing technique. In cases of vitreous herniation into the anterior chamber, the pushing of the vitreous strand back to the retropupillary space with high molecular weight viscoelastic is necessary.

After the injection of sufficient quantities of viscoelastic into the capsular bag to restore its normal shape, a curved needle carrying a looped 10-0 Prolene (polypropylene) is inserted through the anterior chamber and passed along the back surface of the anterior capsule to pierce the equator of the capsular bag before penetrating ciliary sulcus and sclera (Fig. 12–32). Procedures following the penetration of the capsular bag by the suture must be performed with great care so as not to induce a capsular tear from the point of penetration. IOL insertion is performed bimanually to avoid excessive stress to the lens capsule (Fig. 12–33), and the viscoelastic is removed, as gently as possible, with a Simcoe cannula.

The advantage of sutured in-the-bag IOLs is that the shape of the lens capsule can be

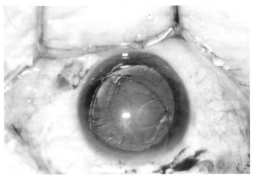

FIGURE 12—30. Zonular dehiscence greater than 120 degrees.

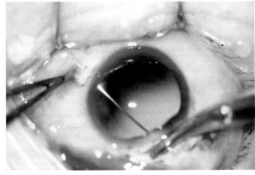

FIGURE 12—32. A 10-0 prolene suture is used for suturing the bag to the sclera.

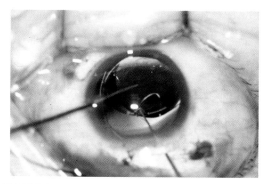

FIGURE 12—33. Bimanual IOL insertion.

almost perfectly maintained, forming a septum between the anterior chamber and the vitreous cavity. Once the IOL is sutured in place, the capsular bag is fully extended by the haptics, and the anterior chamber and vitreous cavity are completely separated by the lens capsule. This means that after the fixation suture is ligated, there is virtually no risk of vitreous herniation and complicated vitreous treatment is not necessary (Fig. 12–34).

The disadvantage of the technique is that the cataract extraction itself is very complex. Also, in cases with more than 120 degrees of zonular dehiscence or cases of cataracts with weak zonulae in all directions, it is very difficult to keep the lens capsule intact without the capsular tension ring. Another potential disadvantage is the risk of capsular rupture induced by the needle penetration.

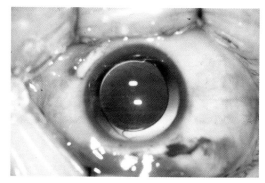

FIGURE 12—34. Surgery completed without vitreous herniation.

■ Tips and Pearls

1. Cataract surgery in presence of a mild zonular dehiscence (less than 3 clock hours), can be managed by conventional phacoemulsification surgery.
2. In presence of a moderate zonular disinsertion (3–5 clock hours), insertion of an endocapsular ring will be required for a safe lensectomy or cataract surgery.
3. When the subluxation involves up to 7 clock hours, you may decide to perform scleral fixation of the capsular bag or the technique of insertion of the capsular ring along with in-the-bag capsule-IOL scleral fixation.
4. For extremely loose cataracts, intracapsular cataract extraction will be required followed by insertion of an anterior chamber IOL or a scleral-fixated posterior chamber lens if the former is not indicated.
5. In the presence of a subluxated cataract, the incision is made at the central axis and location of the remaining intact zonules.
6. Capsular rings of 10 mm in diameter are the most commonly used and are indicated in patients with normal axial length. The 11 mm in diameter rings are indicated when mild and moderate myopia is present. The 12 mm endocapsular ring is reserved for the high myopic patients.
7. The capsular rings are indicated in the prevention of capsular contraction, intraoperative zonular disinsertion, and to help provide pseudophakia in subluxated lenses.
8. You should consider the use of the endocapsular ring for all cases of zonular dehiscence of more than 3 clock hours except in extremely loose lenses.
9. IOL insertion should be performed as gently and carefully as possible to avoid further zonular disinsertion or, a capsular tear caused by the suture should the scleral fixation of the capsule alone or capsule-IOL technique had been performed.
10. In mature cataracts, the capsular bag

might not be strong enough to withstand the suture fixation technique.

REFERENCES

1. Cionni R, Osher R. Endocapsular ring approach to the subluxated cataractous lens. J Cataract Refract Surg 1995;21:245-249.
2. Tokuda Y. IOL in-the-bag suture is a new approach to zonular dehiscence. Ocular Surg News 1997;15(2):19.
3. Morcher GmbH. Kapuzinerweg 12. D- 70374; Stuttgart, Germany.
4. Corneal Paris. 76 Avenue Saint Mandé. 075012 Paris. France.
5. Witchel B, Legler UFL. New approaches to zonular cases: the capsular ring. Audiovisual J Cataract Implant Surg 1993;9(4).

13

Phacoemulsification in Intumescent and Rock Hard Cataracts

ABHAY R. VASAVADA, JOSE A. CLAROS, AND RAMINDER SINGH

This chapter highlights the special features of two very challenging cataracts for a phacosurgeon. Both of these demand good planning and appropriate strategy to achieve a consistently successful outcome. In some parts of the world where patients present themselves with long standing advanced cataracts, the surgeon has to be proficient in dealing with rock-hard as well as intumescent cataracts as they often coexist. The major areas of difficulty they pose are ensuring a strong continuous opening in the anterior capsule, and safe removal of the cataract.

■ Phacoemulsification in Intumescent Cataracts

The intumescent cataract is mainly observed in two forms. In certain cases the cortex is liquefied with a central hard nucleus, leading to a morgagnian cataract. In other cases, hydration of lens fibers takes place but the cortex does not get totally liquefied. The lens size increases and the cataract becomes intumescent. It is the latter type that we would like to focus on.

Special Problems with Intumescent Cataracts

Intumescent mature cataracts have always posed a challenge for phacoemulsification. Careful planning and utmost skill are required. It is very difficult to ensure a continuous capsulorhexis. Nuclei of varying hardness may be camouflaged by the totally opaque cortex. A hard nucleus combined with uncertain continuity of the rhexis margin leads to an unpredictable intraoperative course. Often inspite of a successful phacoemulsification, a plaque on the posterior capsule or residual posterior capsular opacification (PCO) disappoints the surgeon and the patient.

Why Rhexis is Difficult to Perform in Intumescent Cataracts

The difficulty in performing capsulorhexis arises because of two major factors: poor visibility and raised intracapsular pressure.

Poor Visibility

There is absence of the red glow. The liquefied lens content oozes out immediately as the capsule is punctured. This can be washed with balanced salt solution (BSS).[1] However, fluid can flow into the capsular bag and increase the pressure within it. This can cause the tear to extend to the periphery. We suggest replacing the fluid by viscoelastic to maintain clarity and keep the anterior chamber deep (Fig. 13–1).

Raised Intracapsular Pressure

Raised intracapsular pressure arises from the intumescence of the lens fibers and is a major detrimental factor. With intumescence, shallowing of the anterior chamber is more in the center than at the periphery as a result of the convex anterior capsular dome. In cataracts where the lens fibers have liquefied, the lens milk oozes out and the intracapsular pressure is reduced with the initial puncture. Consequently, it becomes less difficult to perform the capsulorhexis. In intumescent cataracts where the lens fibers have not totally liquefied, this does not happen. The intracapsular pressure persists even after the initial puncture is made. Consequently, it becomes difficult to control the capsulorhexis, and the tear tends to extend to the periphery.

Strategy for the Capsulorhexis

The accepted recommendations to aid capsulorhexis include dimming the operating room lights, increasing the operating microscope magnification and coaxial illumination, and the routine use of a viscoelastic material. The use of diathermy, endoilluminator, vitrector, scissors, and staining of the lens capsule have also been suggested.[2-6]

In intumescent mature cataracts, a continuous curvilinear capsulorhexis (CCC) can be consistently achieved by aiming for a small opening. A small capsulorhexis, however, may be associated with anterior capsule opacification, capsular contraction syndrome, and capsular bag hyperdistension syndrome.[7] The solution is to enlarge the capsulorhexis after phacoemulsification known as the two stage approach.[8] This approach combined with our own method of enlargement of rhexis has allowed us to achieve a continuous rhexis with increased consistency.[9]

Initial Small Rhexis

The anterior chamber is filled with high viscosity sodium hyaluronate (Healon GV^R). This flattens the convex anterior capsular dome and relaxes the zonules to some extent. One should aim for a 3 to 4 mm rhexis (Fig. 13–2). The success rate with such a rhexis technique is high for the following obvious reasons:[10] You are away from the periphery and have a greater safety margin when the tear tends to go peripherally; the central zone is free from zonules, which tend to direct the tear to the periphery; and the flattening of the anterior capsule dome produced by the high viscosity viscoelastic is at greater at the center of the field.

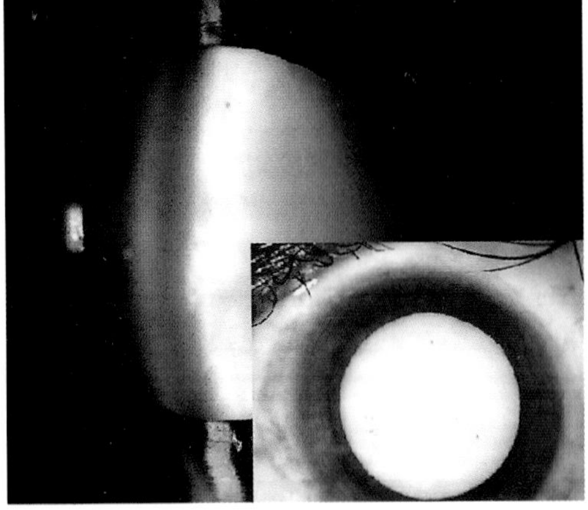

FIGURE 13–1. Total white cataract.

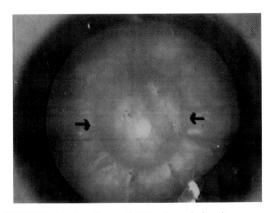

FIGURE 13–2. A small (3 to 4 mm) rhexis.

Enlarging the Initial Capsulorhexis

The capsular bag, with the small capsulorhexis and the anterior chamber are filled with viscoelastic. The viscoelastic must be injected within the bag to push the posterior capsule backwards. An iris spatula is introduced through the side port incision and is placed immediately underneath the anterior capsule. The cystotome needle is introduced through the main incision and placed on the iris spatula (Fig. 13–3). A gentle touch and slight travel on the spatula toward the margin of the capsulorhexis create a break in its continuity. Unlike the sharp cut produced by scissors, this maneuver results in an irregular multi-puncture-like cut. The needle and iris spatula are withdrawn. A pair of capsulorhexis forceps is used to grasp the tear and convert it into a flap, which is slowly maneuvered around, enlarging the original opening. In the process the flap is regrasped several times. If the surgeon desires to break the continuity of the rhexis at the subincisional margin, a curved hook like a chopper can be used. Once the enlargement is achieved, additional cortical cleanup can be performed. An intraocular lens (IOL) is then implanted in the bag.

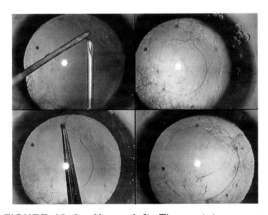

FIGURE 13–3. Upper left: The cystotome needle is placed on the iris spatula, which supports the anterior capsule and protects the posterior capsule. **Upper right:** Irregular, multi-puncture-like cut produced by the cystotome. **Lower left:** The flap is grasped and regrasped. **Lower right:** The enlarged capsulorhexis.

Adaptation for the Phacoemulsification Technique

Once the small size rhexis is achieved, no attempt should be made to hydrodissect or delineate the cataract. In soft cataracts, lens removal does not pose any special problems. However, we often get a nuclear surprise and encounter nuclei of varying hardness. One should therefore develop the skill to deal with a hard cataract through a small rhexis.

For rock-hard cataracts, the technique of step-by-step, chop in situ and separation, helps to divide the cataract in multiple small pieces.[11] Repeated chopping and stuffing enables us to consume the lens fragments in a controlled way by reducing the energy required and maintaining a low aspiration flow rate (18 cc/minute).[12] Stuffing allows us to keep preset vacuum at a low level, which in turn would reduce the surge.

A Study of White Mature Cataracts

We conducted a prospective clinical study of 60 patients with white mature cataracts who underwent phacoemulsification at Iladevi Cataract & IOL Research Centre (Ahmedabad, India) between June 1 and December 15, 1995.[10] The average age of the patients was 54 years (range of 39 to 73 years). Our sample included 36 males and 24 females.

Anterior Chamber Depth

The average anterior chamber depth was 2.6 mm. Seventeen patients (28%) had an anterior chamber depth of less than 2.2 mm.

Capsulorhexis

Continuous capsulorhexis was achieved in 57 eyes (95%). The size of the rhexis achieved initially was 3.8 mm (range 3.5 to 5.1). Enlargement of the capsulorhexis was felt necessary in 29 eyes (48%). The capsulotomy size at the end of the surgery was 5.6 mm (range 4 to 6.5). None of the eyes developed uncontrolled peripheral extension during enlargement of the rhexis.

Intracapsular Pressure

Intracapsular pressure was judged to be raised in 24 eyes (40%). Out of these, continuous

Table 13–1. Capsulorhexis and Intracapsular Pressure.

	Complete	Incomplete rhesis	Total
Raised intracapsular pressure	21	3	24
Normal intracapsular pressure	36	0	36
Total	57	3	60

$X2 = 4.74$, $P < .05$, significant. Fisher's Exact Test $p = .0591$.

rhexis was accomplished in only 21 eyes (88%). The raised intracapsular pressure is a significant factor (See Table 13–1).

Grade of Hardness

Fifty percent of the nuclei were graded to be of Grade V hardness. The conditions of the posterior capsule are rated as follows: Plaque, 20 (33%); Residual cortex, 15 (25%); and Clear, 25 (42%).

■ Conclusion

If a continuous capsulorhexis can be achieved, the results of white cataract phacoemulsification are comparable to those of standard cataract surgery. There is an increased possibility of finding a plaque or a posterior capsule opacification intraoperatively. We recommend the use of high viscosity sodium hyaluronate for performing the capsulorhexis. We endorse the two-stage capsulorhexis approach. However, one should be prepared to deal with a hard cataract through a small rhexis. Our technique of enlargement is simple, precise, and safe.

■ Phacoemulsification in Rock Hard Cataracts

Phacoemulsification in a rock hard cataract is a different proposition altogether. The black cataract poses a unique challenge to a phacosurgeon (Fig. 13–4). The extraordinarily tough cataract tests all the skills and experience of the surgeon. The incidence of intra- and postoperative complications remains high in the hands of surgeons who have to deal with such an entity only occasionally in their practice. It is important to estimate the lens hardness preoperatively and be prepared with an appropriate strategy.

Some varieties of hard cataract do not seem to fall within the current lens hardness grading system. In our part of the world, we routinely have to face black and brunescent cataracts. Understanding the peculiar difficulties in dealing with rock hard cataracts and the adaptation necessary in the surgical technique are important for achieving an outcome comparable to standard cataract phacoemulsification.

Difficulties with Rock Hard Cataracts

Poor Visibility

There is usually little or no glow because of the dense cataract. This makes capsulorhexis difficult to perform.

Capsular Changes

The anterior capsule is fragile and fractures easily. At times a plaque formation on the an-

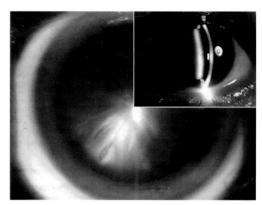

FIGURE 13–4. Black cataract. Note silver gray shine.

terior capsule is found. This can be in the form of small or big patches.

Large Lens Size
A large lens reduces the depth of the anterior chamber as well as the working space. It also expands the capsular bag and puts it on stretch. Excessive manipulation during the hydrodivision procedure increases the risk of posterior capsule rupture. This also makes rotation a tricky procedure.

Cortico-Capsular Adhesion
This is frequently observed in long-standing hard cataracts. This resists free rotation of the nucleus.

Epinucleus
The compactness of fibers blocks hydrodelineation in most cases. This prevents the creation of the epinucleus shell. Hence, the phacoable nucleus remains quite large and there is minimal mechanical cushion effect.

Peculiarities of the Lens Fibers
The fibers in advanced hard cataracts are very cohesive and tenacious, commonly described as leathery fibers.[11] These fibers seem to "absorb" phacoenergy. They resist all the conventional methods of division. Even a few fibers can keep the entire nucleus in a cohesive form like petals of a flower. This makes phacoemulsification in the bag extremely difficult and risky. Forceful attempts for division of nucleus and the need to keep the power, aspiration flow rate, and vacuum at higher setting, increase the risk to the capsular-zonular apparatus. The phaco energy consumption in such cases is much higher than the standard phacoemulsification. There is also an increased risk of hard fragments coming in close contact with the endothelium. These can lead to increased endothelial damage.

Special Considerations in the Surgical Technique

Anesthesia
A hard cataract can take a long time for removal. Peribulbar anesthesia is more desirable than topical anesthesia in such cases, until the surgeon achieves consistency.

Incisional Burns
There is an increased incidence of incisional burns during emulsification of hard cataracts because of the prolonged phaco energy consumption.[13] This risk can be reduced by adopting the temporal approach, placing a corneal incision, making a wider incision, keeping a high aspiration flow rate, and using special sleeves and tips (tapered sleeves[R], microflow tips[R], and microseal tips[R]). The temporal approach reduces the angulation between the incision bed and the phacotip by avoiding the brow ridge. A clear corneal tunnel is shorter than a scleral tunnel, implying less tissue contact and less distortion of the incision. A wider incisional tunnel is desirable to allow fluid leakage which helps in cooling the phacoemulsification tip. With high aspiration flow rate, the cooling of the tip is achieved faster. A microtip with a tapered sleeve (Legacy[R]) maintains better irrigation fluid around the phacotip. Dr. Graham Barrett's microflow fluted tip also helps to keep an effective fluid cushion through small incision. The Mackool system, with its special double sleeve, is an excellent way of reducing incisional burn for a tight incision.

Viscoelastics
Dispersive viscoelastics as the chondroitin sulphate or methyl cellulose, are desirable during the lens removal. For capsulorhexis and IOL implantation, a cohesive viscoelastic as sodium hyaluronate, is preferred. For patients with compromised endothelium in an eye with rock hard cataracts, we prefer dispersive viscoelastics every minute of the procedure which we call "one minute phacoemulsification".

Capsulorhexis
A small capsulorhexis holds the hard lens fragment within the capsular bag better than a large one. Moreover, an attempt to achieve an initial large rhexis could lead to an uncontrolled peripheral extension due to poor visibility and enlarged lens size. The capsulorhexis should be enlarged after the completion of

phacoemulsification but before the IOL implantation. This two-stage approach facilitates endophacoemulsification and reduces anterior capsular opacification by leaving behind a small area of anterior capsule.

Hydrodissection

We perform cortical-cleaving hydrodissection.[14] It is achieved by tenting up the anterior capsule with the help of a 26 gauge cannula and injecting fluid just under the anterior capsule, near the lens equator. But care should be taken not to tent up the anterior capsule too much because of the increased volume of the cataract. Hydrodissection should be gentle and not forceful. Excessive injection should be avoided. Because of the density of the nucleus, the fluid wave traveling behind the lens is not visible. Sometimes the forward movement of the nucleus takes place suggesting an effective separation of cataract from capsule. In effective hydrodissection, the capsulorhexis opening becomes more prominent and readily visible.

Hydrodelineation

In rock-hard cataracts, as a rule, it is extremely difficult to achieve delineation. There is a danger of overdoing the procedure and producing stress to the capsular bag and zonules.

Rotation

Long-standing cataracts, black cataracts, and some mixed cataracts with cortical opacities tend to have cortico-capsular adhesions. These adhesions resist free rotation. They should be anticipated and multiple cortical-cleaving hydrodissection with a curved cannula should be attempted. Forceful attempts to rotate should be avoided.

Sculpting

The anterior chamber is filled with dispersive viscoelastic. The Kelman tip has an advantage. Its 20-degree bent makes it more effective than the straight tips. It is also less traumatic to the superior capsular bag and zonules while trying to sculpt very deep into the nucleus. Bevel down sculpting is also a useful technique to minimize endothelial damage. Keeping the bevel down makes phacoemulsification more effective and reduces energy requirements. Many surgeons find the 45 degrees phaco tip more useful. Should you choose a 45 degrees tip during the sculpting stage, it may become necessary to change to a 30 degrees tip for easier occlusion at a later stage of the procedure. Down slope sculpting as suggested by Gimbel is a good technique.[15] However, extreme care should be taken to reduce the stress on the superior capsular bag and zonules. Suggested parameters for sculpting are surgeon controlled power at 100%, aspiration flow rate of 25 cc per min and, vacuum of 40 mmHg.

Trench vs. Crater

Adequate space in the center should be created. In the hard cataract it is safer to create a large space. A crater is preferred over the trench as it gives enough central space for maneuvering the divided fragments (Fig. 13–5). An attempt to divide and manipulate the lens fragments without a central space is difficult because of closeness of fragments in a crowded space and can lead to capsular bag distortion.[16] Therefore, *creation of central space is very critical.*

Nuclear Division

There are many innovative techniques to deal with hard cataracts. In Shepherd's in situ fracture technique, the nucleus is divided into four quadrants.[17] Gimbel described the divide and conquer nucleofractis.[18] Fine and his co-authors described a crack and flip combination.[19] In these techniques the division and separation of the nucleus is achieved by out-

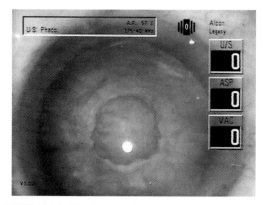

FIGURE 13–5. A crater in a brown black cataract.

ward separation. A forced separation may produce stress on the capsular bag and zonules. This outward separation is not needed in the Nagahara's phaco chop.[20] This was modified to Stop and Chop by Koch and coauthors.[16] However, even with the chop action it is not always possible to achieve a complete division of the nucleus in extremely hard leathery cataracts.

We describe our approach, which involves the judicious combination of step by step chop in situ and lateral separating movements.[11] This has helped us to sever the leathery fibers completely and achieve multiple small lens fragments. *Creation of multiple small fragments is the essence for successful outcome.*

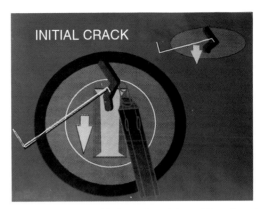

FIGURE 13-6. Initial crack achieved by chop in situ.

Step-by-Step Chop In Situ and Lateral Separation

The step-by-step chop in situ and lateral separation method is carried out in the following sequence:

Vacuum Seal.

The machine settings are changed to 80% power, aspiration flow rate 18 cc/min and vacuum to 200 to 400 mmHg. The phaco tip is buried at 6 o'clock to produce a vacuum seal. This results in an effective hold on the nucleus.

Chop In Situ.

The chopper is placed adjacent to the impaled phaco tip. The vertical element of the chopper is depressed posteriorly (towards the optic nerve) (Fig. 13-6). This produces a crack. The chopper remains within the capsulorhexis and is never placed underneath the anterior capsule beyond the rhexis margin. There is no risk of zonulolysis or capsular tear. This is quite different from the conventional phacochop maneuver.

Lateral Separation.

In hard cataracts, the initial crack seldom reaches the bottom. The chopper is repositioned in the depths of the crack and pushed laterally. The lateral separating movement extends the crack to the bottom and severs the leathery fibers holding the nucleus halves together. The two hemisections are produced in a gradual step-by-step fashion by repeated lateral movements of the chopper at different sites all along the bottom of the trench or crater, while the phacoprobe still holds the nucleus steady at 6 o'clock (Fig. 13-7). Each nucleus half is rotated to lie horizontally across the inferior capsular bag. A similar chop in situ and lateral separating movements result into multiple small lens fragments in each hemisection. In dealing with extremely tenacious fibers, outward separation movements by a chopper placed in the depth of the crack produces slight tilting of the fragment (Fig. 13-8). Therefore, this should be done only during the later stages when the capsular bag is partially empty and enough space is available. The newer generation of phaco units enables the surgeon to achieve an appro-

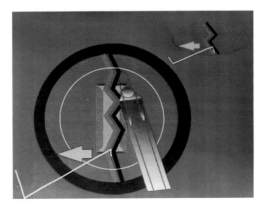

FIGURE 13-7. Complete division into two hemisections.

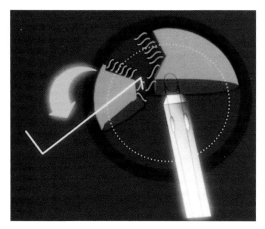

FIGURE 13–8. Notice the chopper severing the fibers in step-by-step fashion. Notice the tilt given to the chopped fragment. Capsular bag is partially empty.

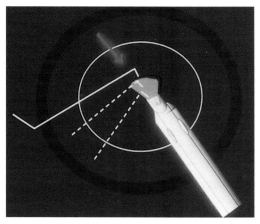

FIGURE 13–10. The small pieces are brought near the port and stuffed mechanically into the lumen of the probe. The foot pedal remains in position 2.

priate level of vacuum and fluidic control (Fig. 13–9).

Removal of Lens Fragments

We recommend the "Chop, Chop and Stuff technique".[12] It is very crucial that fragments are small. Larger fragments as sometimes seen in the four-quadrant technique are difficult to manage and may come in contact with endothelium. The left hand continues chopping (Fig. 13–10), dividing the large fragment into multiple small pieces. The chopper brings the small pieces to the port and stuffs them into the lumen of the port. The high vacuum inside the probe aspirates the small pieces. Little phaco energy is used (at the maximum of 10 to 30% power). The left hand remains in action throughout the procedure.

Table 13–2. Study of Rock Hard Cataracts

INCISION
  A corneal tunnel was fashioned in 25 cases.
CAPSULORHEXIS
  Complete capsulorhexis was achieved in all the cases. The initial small rhexis was enlarged in 7 (18%) cases.
HYDRODELINEATION
  Was achieved only in 8 (20%) patients.
ROTATION
  Was not achieved in 8 (20%) patients.
PHACOENERGY
  Average energy dissipated during sculpting = 1.32 + 0.24 CDE.
  Average total dissipated energy = 2.19 + 0.44 cumulative dissipated energy (CDE). It is interesting to note here that 60% of total energy was used during sculpting.
INCISIONAL BURNS
  Eight (20%) patients developed incisional burns of mild to moderate degree.
CORNEAL EVALUATION
  Mean corneal thickness increased by 22.2% on the first postoperative day. Corneal thickness returned to normal between the first and third month.
  At the end of one year, endothelial cell density decreased by 13.12%, the coefficient of variation increased by 10.20% and in hexagonality decreased by 20.30%.

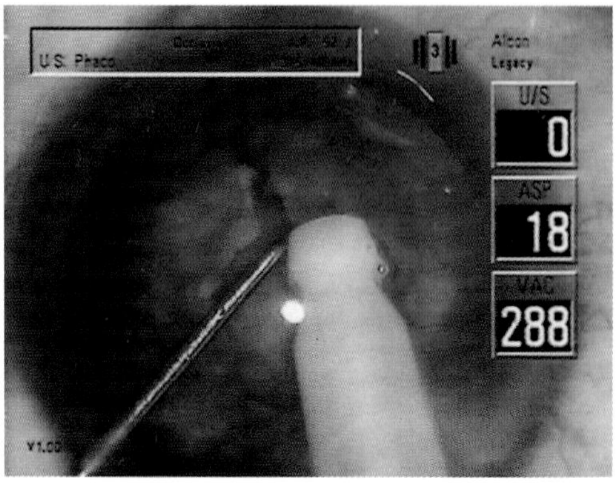

FIGURE 13–9. Chop in situ. Notice zero US power and high vacuum levels.

Rock Hard Cataract Study

A prospective randomized controlled study of 40 patients with grade five and five plus cataract conducted from January 1996 to February 1997 at Iladevi Cataract & IOL Research Centre is briefly sumarized in Table 13–2.

■ Conclusion

The rock hard cataract demands appropriate strategy and planning. Obtaining multiple small fragments is the essence of a successful outcome. Creation of central space is crucial. Bevel down, "step-by-step chop in situ and separation" and "stop chop, chop and stuff" are useful techniques for safe removal of fragments. The ultimate outcome is comparable to that of standard cataract phacoemulsification.

■ Tips and Pearls

For Intumescent Cataracts

1. Perform the continuous curvilinear capsulotomy (CCC) under dim operating room illumination, high magnification, and under high viscosity viscoelastic material.
2. Aim for a small opening. You can always enlarge it later. We suggest the two-stage capsulorhexis approach.
3. Do not attempt to hydrodissect or hydrodelineate after the small CCC has been achieved.
4. You may find a very hard nucleus in 50% of the times. The hardness may be camouflaged by the totally opaque cortex. Be prepared to deal with a hard cataract through a small rhexis.
5. There is an increased possibility of finding a plaque or posterior capsular opacification intraoperatively (33%).

For Rock Hard Cataracts

1. Remember the difficulties in dealing with these type of cataracts: poor visibility, capsular changes, large lens size, cortico-capsular adhesions, scarce epinucleus, and the peculiar lens fibers present.
2. Peribulbar anesthesia may be more desirable than topical.
3. Avoid incisional burns, make the right incision, choose the correct tip, and use high aspiration flow rate for sculpting. Most of the phaco energy will go during this stage of the procedure.
4. Use the appropriate viscoelastic material during the different steps of the procedure.
5. Avoid a very large capsulorhexis opening, perform a gentle hydrodissection, and avoid forceful attempts to rotate the nucleus.
6. In rock hard cataracts, creation of a central space is critical. The creation of multiple small fragments is the essence of the successful outcome.
7. The techniques of "step-by-step chop in situ and separation" and "stop and chop, chop and stuff" are very useful for the safe removal of nuclear fragments.

REFERENCES

1. Gimbel HV, Willerscheidt AB. What to do with limited view: the intumescent cataract. J Cataract Refract Surg 1993;19:657–661.
2. Hausmann N, Richard G. Investigations on diathermy for anterior capsulotomy. Invest OphthalmVisual Sci 1991;32:2155–2159.
3. Mansour AM. Anterior capsulorhexis in hypermature cataract. J Cataract Refract Surg 1993;19:116–117.
4. Vajpayee RS, Angra SK, Honavar SG, et al. Capsulotomy for phacoemulsification in hypermature cataract. J Cataract Refract Surg 1995;21:612–615.
5. Hoffer KJ, Mcfarland JE. Intracameral subcapsular fluoreccin staining for improved visualization during capsulorhexis in mature cataracts (letter). J Cataract Refract Surg 1993;19:566.
6. Cimetta DJ, Gatti M, Libianco G. Haemocoloration of the anterior capsule in white cataract CCC. Eur J Implant Ref Surg 1995;7:184–185.
7. Davison JA. Capsule contraction syndrome. J Cataract Refract Surg 1993;19:582–589.
8. Gimbel HV. Two-stage capsulorhexis for endocapsular phacoemulsification. J Cataract Refract Surg 1990;16:246–249.
9. Vasavada AR, Desai J, Singh R. Enlarging the capsulorhexis. J Cataract Refract Surg 1997;23:329–331.
10. Vasavada A, Singh R, Desai J. Phacoemulsification in

white mature cataracts. J Cataract Refract Surg 1998; 24:270–277.
11. Vasavada AR, Singh R, Desai J. Step-by-step chop in situ and separation of very dense cataracts. J Cataract Refract Surg 1998;24:156–159.
12. Vasavada AR, Desai JP. Stop, chop, chop, and stuff. J Cataract Refract Surg 1996;22:526–529.
13. Wirt H, Heisler JM, Domrus DV. Phacoburns: experimental study for evaluation of risk factors. Eur J Implant Refract Surg 1995;7:275–278.
14. Fine IH. Cortical cleaving hydrodissection. J Cataract Refract Surg 1992;18:508–512.
15. Gimbel HV. Down slope sculpting. J Cataract Refract Surg 1992;18:614–618.
16. Koch PS, Katzen LE. Stop and chop phacoemulsification. J Cataract Refract Surg 1994;20:566–570.
17. Shepherd JR. In situ fracture. J Cataract Refractive Surg 1990;16:436–440.
18. Gimbel HV. Divide and conquer nucleofractis phacoemulsification. Development and variations. J Cataract Refract Surg 1991;17:281–291.
19. Fine HI, Maloney WF, Dillman DM. Crack and flip phacoemulsification technique. J Cataract Refract Surg 1993;19:797–802.
20. Nagahara K. Phaco-Chop. Film presented at the 3rd American-International Congress on Cataract, IOL, and Refractive Surgery. Seattle, WA, May 1993.

14

Phacoemulsification in Posterior Polar Developmental Cataracts

ABHAY R. VASAVADA AND RAMINDER SINGH

Posterior polar cataract presents a special challenge to the phacosurgeon in that it is known to have a predisposition to posterior capsular dehiscence during cataract surgery.[1] It is an important type of congenital cataract which affects vision early in its course. The lens is usually clear at birth and the cataractous changes take place later in life, usually in the thirties or the forties. The white dense opacity is located near the nodal point of the eye in the central axis.

■ Incidence

The incidence of posterior polar cataract is reported as 4 in 1000 cases by Dr. Lucio Buratto.[2] Our own retrospective search of outpatient records revealed an incidence of 8 in 1000 cataract patients.

■ Forms

The posterior polar cataract may occur in two forms[3]: stationary and progressive.

Stationary is a well limited circular white opacity located on the central posterior capsule. The concentric thickened rings around the central plaque opacity gives an appearance of a bull's eye (Fig. 14–1). This form is the most commonly seen.

Progressive changes take place in the posterior cortex in the form of radiating "rider" opacities (Fig. 14–2). These opacities do not involve the nucleus.

Sometimes there is a smaller satellite rosette lesion adjacent to the central opacity. Although it is reported to be associated with a remnant of the hyaloid artery or mesodermal tissue, we have never seen this association.[4,5] Occassionally we have seen formations like oil droplets in the surrounding area. Very rarely will a preexisting tear in the posterior capsule be visible. The presence of dense white spots adjacent to the "onion ring" cataract as a sure sign of posterior capsular dehiscence has been described.[6] In elderly patients the posterior polar cataract may be camouflaged by nuclear sclerosis and at times the diagnosis is missed during the preoperative evaluation (Fig. 14–3).

■ Symptoms

The stationary form of posterior polar cataract is compatible with good visual acuity. Normally, the patient seeks help in his or her thir-

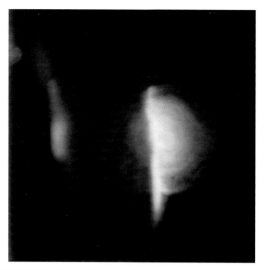

FIGURE 14–1. Classical whorl opacity giving rise to bull's eye appearance.

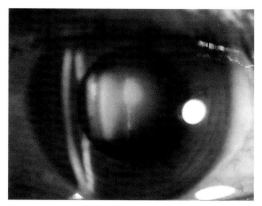

FIGURE 14–3. Age related nuclear sclerosis camouflaging the posterior polar cataract.

ties or forties. The common symptom is intolerance to light. Glare affects the patient most severely when the source of light is close to the object of vision. For instance, night driving becomes difficult. Forward light scattering (light scattering towards retina) accounts for glare as well as for reduced contrast sensitivity and visual acuity.[7] The symptoms worsen with development of cortical rider opacities. However, in our experience, patients with the stationary form of cataract also complain of increasing visual symptoms. We have so far failed to observe any detectable progressive change in these patients.

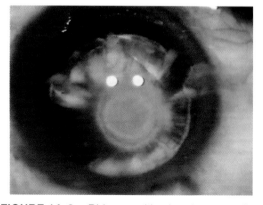

FIGURE 14–2. Rider opacities in a long standing posterior polar cataract in a 72-year-old female.

■ Genetics

Posterior polar cataract is usually inherited as autosomal dominant.[8,9] Sporadic cases may represent a mutation.[10] The majority are bilateral. Reported pedigrees are associated with a variety of systemic and ocular conditions. However, such associations in clinical practice are very rare. The gene for posterior polar cataract has been linked with the haptoglobin locus on chromosome 16.[11]

Light and electronmicroscopy of plaque posterior subcapsular opacity have been documented by Dark and Streeten[12] and Eshagian et al.[13,14] The major change is the breakdown of the normally regular parallel rows of lens fibers into rounded globules. Membranous whorls or myelin figures are a common finding. Plaque opacity is more cortical than vacuolar posterior subcapsular opacity of other etiology.[15]

■ Pathogenesis

The pathogenesis of posterior polar cataract is unknown. It is speculated that it is caused by the persistence of the hyaloid artery or invasion of the lens by mesoblastic tissue.[4,5] There is little clinical evidence in the majority of cases. It is our speculation that the aberrant epithelial cells from the equator find their way to the posterior pole, undergo pseudometaplasia and form a dense opacity. The continuation of this process leads to encapsulation of the original opacity, giving rise to concentric rings and whorl appearance.

■ Predisposition to Rupture

The posterior capsule has an inherent weakness and therefore is predisposed to rupture.[1] There is no histopathological consensus among investigators on the thinness of the posterior capsule. The plaque could be adherent to the posterior capsule. During epinucleus removal, the plaque does not detach from the posterior capsule which eventually ruptures. Therefore, the shape of the posterior capsular rupture is not always circular. The configuration of the posterior capsular defect depends on the exact genesis of a specific cataract and the traction applied to the plaque during surgery. Among cases where the posterior capsule remains intact, we have sometimes observed a thin posterior capsule and, on other occasions, patchy plaque-like opacification. Osher et al. reported 26% incidence of posterior capsule rupture in their series of 31 cases.[1]

■ Management

Removal of the posterior developmental cataract should be delayed as long as possible. Surgery should be considered only when the patient finds it very difficult to carry out his or her important activities. The patient should be informed of the possibility of intraoperative posterior capsule rupture and consequences of vitreous loss. We also discuss the various possible fixation sites for intraocular lens and also warn the patient that in rare events it could become difficult to fixate an intraocular lens (IOL) safely. In cases compounded by advanced nuclear sclerosis, the possibility of dropped fragment should also be brought to the patient's attention.

In our opinion, phacoemulsification is preferred over conventional ECCE, because the former gives better control with closed chamber techniques. However, the phacosurgeon should anticipate events and plan the relevant strategy for every step of the surgery.

Anesthesia

"Injection" anesthesia is desirable and should be preferred over its topical counterpart. In the event of posterior capsular rupture, the operation time may be prolonged. Therefore, our preference is for peribulbar anesthesia. We also apply intermittent oculorbital compression (super pinky) to achieve ocular hypotony. This may reduce the vitreous pressure.

Incision

We create a main corneal valve incision appropriate for a foldable IOL, and two paracentesis incisions. Following the initial entry into the anterior chamber, viscoelastic is injected before further incisions are fashioned. The viscoelastic prevents shallowing of the anterior chamber and scleral collapse. This is especially important for young patients who have low scleral rigidity.

Anterior Capsulorhexis

The optimal size of this opening is 4 to 5 mm. Too large an opening may not give adequate support for sulcus fixated IOL and will not be able to capture the optic. Too small an opening may increase the hydrostatic pressure in the capsular bag during hydrodelineation and it may also make the lens removal difficult. The procedure is performed very slowly with a 26 gauge needle or with a capsulorhexis forceps under viscoelastic material.

Hydrodissection

Hydrodissection means injecting BSS right underneath the anterior capsule and separating the entire cataract from the capsular bag. The fluid wave traveling behind the lens is a sign of complete separation of the cataract from the capsule. Cortico capsular cleaving hydrodissection is very useful in standard cataract phacoemulsification.[16] However it *should not be attempted in a posterior polar cataract* as it can precipitate posterior capsule rupture.

Hydrodelineation

It means injecting BSS in the substance of the cataract. This reduces the volume of the nucleus and produces a mechanical cushion effect of epinucleus (Fig. 14–4). This in turn reduces the possibility of capsular rupture during nucleus removal. *We regard hydrodelineation as mandatory in such a cataract.* Efforts should be made to generate a thick epinucleus to protect the capsule during phacoemulsification.

Rotation

An attempt to rotate the nucleus can lead to capsule rupture. During the nucleus removal stage, a gentle rotation of a well delineated central nucleus may be tried if it is unavoidable.

Nucleus Removal

Maximum stress to the capsule bag takes place during emulsification of the nucleus. All techniques at this stage should be geared to facilitate the removal of nucleus inside the bag, within the cushion effect of the epinucleus (Fig. 14–5). Biannual cracking and division of the nucleus involving outward movements can result in distortion of the capsular bag.

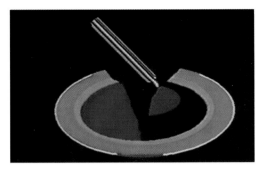

FIGURE 14–5. Chopped fragment is emulsified within the cushion of epinucleus.

A central space is created by sculpting a trench. The trench does not extend beyond the capsulorhexis margin. The power setting is kept at a slightly higher scale to reduce any inadvertent mechanical movement of the nucleus by the phacoprobe. Suggested settings for sculpting are 60 to 70% of power, 0 mmHg of vacuum, and an aspiration flow rate of 25 cc/minute. We prefer "chop in situ" action for lens division.[17] The lens is held firmly after achieving adequate occlusion. The vertical element of the chopper is depressed posteriorly (towards optic nerve). The chopper remains in the central area and at no time does it move underneath the anterior capsule. The chopping maneuver is thus repeated to produce multiple small fragments. The lens fragments are removed in the central space by the "stop, chop, chop and stuff" technique.[17] The chopper in the left hand brings the small fragments to the phacotip. This helps us to keep the aspiration flow rate low. Once the fragments are brought to the tip, they are stuffed by the chopper. Smaller fragments are easily stuffed and aspirated at a lower vacuum level. The surge phenomenon is also reduced. At this stage phaco power, aspiration and vacuum should be kept at low levels. The bottle should be at a 50 cm height. Suggested settings are: phacopower at 60%; vacuum 100 to 120 mmHg; and aspiration flow rate 16 to 18 cc/minute. The anterior chamber should consistently remain well formed. Viscoelastic is injected into the anterior chamber before withdrawing the instrument from the eye. This prevents forward movement of posterior capsule and anterior vitreous.

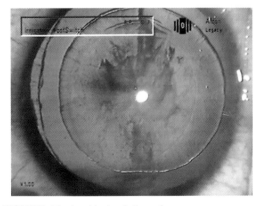

FIGURE 14–4. Hydrodelineation.

Epinucleus Removal

With adequate care and an appropriate technique, it is possible to safely remove the nucleus and leave the epinucleus shell behind. Removing the epinucleus is the dreaded step of the procedure. The central area should be kept attached until the last stage (Fig. 14–6). The epinucleus is stripped off all around the peripheral cortex by using automated irrigation aspiration (I/A). We keep the aspiration flow rate at 20 cc/min with preset vacuum at 400 mmHg. Collapse of the anterior chamber should be avoided by injecting viscoelastic every time before the instrument is withdrawn. Two port I/A, utilizing one port for irrigation and the other for aspiration, gives better control and ensures complete removal of the cortex. Some surgeons prefer manual removal of the epinucleus bowl, using the Simcoe cannula.

If the Posterior Capsule is Ruptured

Careful planning during the earlier stages of the procedure could prevent a rupture. The capsular rupture becomes inevitable in some cases when the central epinucleus is being aspirated along with the plaque opacity. The posterior capsular rupture is typically round with an extension to the periphery (Fig. 14–7). The initial circular dehiscence assumes an oval shape because of vitreous pressure. Once the rupture is recognized, the chamber should be filled with viscoelastic. Two port anterior vitrectomy should be performed for this purpose.

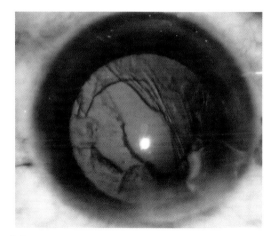

FIGURE 14–7. Peripheral extension of the initial circular posterior capsular dehiscence.

Two Port Anterior Vitrectomy

Anterior vitrectomy is performed by using two ports of entry into the eye (Fig. 14–8). One port is for the irrigation cannula (21 gauge) connected to the infusion bottle. The vitrector is introduced through the second paracentesis. The vitrector and irrigation cannula are exchanged through the ports for adequate vitrectomy. Typical unit settings are: cut rate of 350 cuts/minute, vacuum of 150 mmHg, and aspiration flow rate of 15 cc/minute. With a high cut rate and low vacuum and flow rate we

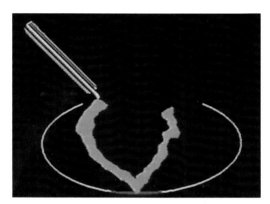

FIGURE 14–6. Central plaque is kept attached until the entire epinucleus is stripped off from the periphery.

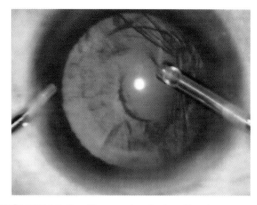

FIGURE 14–8. Two port anterior vitrectomy.

can safely perform the vitrectomy even in areas near the torn capsule.

The objective of the procedure is to perform an adequate central vitrectomy and not a total (peripheral) anterior vitrectomy. Indeed, the vitrector is never placed behind the peripheral posterior capsule. The infusion cannula is directed to the peripheral anterior chamber and the fluid jet is directed towards the angle and away from the defect. This reduces turbulence near the tip of the cutter and avoids further enlargement of the capsular tear. This also reduces hydration of vitreous and forward movement of vitreous into the anterior chamber.[18] At the end an iris spatula is swiped from each port to check for the presence of a vitreous strand caught in the incision.

Cortex Removal

After a vitrectomy is adequately accomplished, the cortex is aspirated using the two port I/A approach. As the irrigation and aspiration probes are exchanged, the entire 360 degree cortex is safely removed. There is no inaccessible subincisional cortex with the two port I/A technique. The remaining capsular support is evaluated for deciding the site for IOL fixation.

Posterior Capsulorhexis

A posterior capsulorhexis may be performed if the rupture is confined to the central area. Dr. Albert Galand reported a successful outcome with posterior capsulorhexis in posterior polar cataract.[19] This should be done after adequate vitrectomy is accomplished and should be performed under high viscosity viscoelastic.

IOL Fixation

The site for haptic placement depends on the extent of the posterior capsular rupture and the integrity of the remaining posterior capsule. If a small central tear is converted into a strong opening by a posterior capsulorhexis, then the IOL is fixated in the capsular bag. It is possible to capture the optic through a small posterior rhexis opening so that the haptics lie in the bag while the optic is behind the posterior capsule.[20] However, in our experience such facility is very rare. More commonly, the posterior capsule tear is large enough to prevent safe placement of the haptics in the bag. In such an event, the haptics are placed in front of the anterior capsule. We have recently been able to capture the optic through an anterior rhexis (Fig. 14–9). We feel that the main advantage of capturing the optic through intact rhexis opening is that it locks the IOL and stabilizes it against the capsular contracting forces.

The Technique for a Foldable IOL

We have recently begun to use the Acrysof (R) IOLs. Since this implant unfolds gradually, the capsular stress is minimized. The slow unfolding also gives control to the surgeon. A high viscosity viscoelastic is injected. The IOL is introduced through the corneal tunnel and is released in front of the anterior capsule. The haptics are then gradually diverted into the bag or the ciliary sulcus depending upon the status of the capsular support. Over the last 2 years we have been successfully implanting foldable acrylic lenses in cases with posterior capsular rupture, including the posterior polar cataract.

When the Posterior Capsule is Intact

In the absence of a posterior capsular rupture, the management is like a standard phacoemulsification. The central capsule should be carefully observed under high magnification. There may be a diffuse central plaque left over the

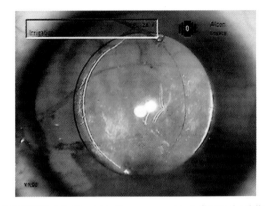

FIGURE 14–9. Haptics are sulcus fixated while optic is captured through an anterior capsulorhexis. Notice the large posterior capsular rupture.

capsule, the central capsule may have scattered areas of small plaque-like residues, or may appear very thin and fragile. Vacuum cleaning of the posterior capsule should be avoided. If required, YAG laser capsulotomy may be performed 3 to 6 months after the surgery.

Removal of Viscoelastic Material

After IOL implantation, the viscoelastic is removed by the two port vitrectomy technique. We use the ATIOP vitrectomy device attached to a Legacy 20000 unit. Here aspiration is preceded by cutting. This technique involves removal of the viscoelastic in a piecemeal and gradual manner. This prevents the drag on the endothelium and sudden collapse of the anterior chamber. High cutting rate with low vacuum and aspiration flow rate facilitate to achieve these objectives.

At the end of the procedure we inject 0.1 ml (1 mg) of vancomycin in the capsular bag. The incisions are left unsutured. Twenty milligrams of garamycin and 2 mg of dexamethasone are injected subconjunctivally. Postoperatively, topical steroid and diclofenac drops are continued for 2 to 3 months. The pupil is kept mobile by cyclopentolate 1% drops every third day for the first 2 weeks. The uveal response, IOP, and retinal status are evaluated carefully.

Camouflaged Opacity

When a dense nuclear sclerosis has camouflaged the posterior polar plaque opacity, it could go unnoticed preoperatively. Then, the posterior capsular rupture could take place at an early stage of the procedure. In such cases, the principles of management remain the same as detailed above. A large sinking fragment should be removed by converting the procedure to manual ECCE. The management of a dropped nucleus should be handled by an experienced vitreoretinal surgeon.

■ Posterior Polar Cataract Study

A prospective clinical study of 22 patients with posterior polar cataracts undergoing phacoemulsification was conducted from December 1995 to May 1997 at the Iladevi Cataract & IOL Research Centre (Ahmedabad, India). The average age of our patients was 56 years (range 22–75 years). Our sample included 13 males and 9 females. Eighteen cases were bilateral while only four were unilateral. The average lens thickness was 3.35 mm as compared to 4.56 mm found in age/sex matched patients with nuclear cataracts attending our clinic. Other varieties of posterior subcapsular cataracts are reported to have similar lens thickness.[21]

The condition of the posterior capsule during surgery was: Rupture, 8 (36%); Plaque, 6 (27%); Clear, 8 (36%).

The Stage at Which Capsular Rupture Occured

In seven cases capsular rupture took place at the time of epinucleus removal, while in one eye it happened while emulsifying the last two fragments.

IOL Fixation

In all 22 eyes we could implant an IOL. In seven of eight cases with rupture, we placed the haptics in the ciliary sulcus. In two of these cases we could capture the optical portion of the IOL through the anterior capsulorhexis. In only one case, the IOL was placed in the bag. The haptics were placed perpendicular to the direction of the capsular rupture.

Follow-up Period

Average 9.5 months (range 3 to 12 months).

Complications

All our patients had a satisfactory outcome at the end of the follow-up period. No patient developed a raised IOP or a retinal break. One patient was detected to have macular edema in the third postoperative week. This was resolved with a topical and systemic nonsteroidal antiinflammatory drugs.

Visual Acuity

Among 22 patients, 14 recorded visual acuity of 20/20 to 20/30. Out of the remaining eight patients, seven gained acuity of 20/40 to 20/60, while one did not improve beyond 20/120, because these patients had a posterior capsular plaque. All the patients with plaque, except two, needed YAG laser capsulotomy. In those patients the vision improved to 20/30.

■ Tips and Pearls

1. Make the patient aware of all possible eventualities.
2. Be ready to manage all possible complications.
3. Hydrodissection is contraindicated but hydrodelineation is mandatory.
4. "Chop in situ," and "chop, chop, and stuff" techniques reduce the stress on the capsular bag.
5. Avoid posterior capsule vacuum cleaning in such eyes.
6. Prevent anterior chamber collapse at every stage of the procedure. Inflate the eye with viscoelastic before withdrawing the instrument.
7. Use every available capsular support for IOL fixation.

REFERENCES

1. Osher RH, Yu BC-4, Koch DD. Posterior polar cataract a predisposition to intraoperative posterior capsule rupture. J Cataract Refract Surg 1990;16:157–167.
2. Lucio B. Consultation section. J Cataract Refract Surg 1994; 20:99–104.
3. Duke-Elder S. Posterior polar cataract. In: Duke-Elder S, (ed). System of Ophthalmology, Vol. III: Normal and Abnormal Development, Congenital Deformities. St Louis: CV Mosby; 1964;723–726.
4. Gifford SR. Congenital anomalies of the lens as seen with the slit lamp. Am J Ophthalmol 1924;7:678–685.
5. Szily AV. The Doyne memorial lecture: the contribution of pathological examinations to the elucidation of the problems of cataract. Trans Ophthalmol Soc UK 1938; 58(2):595–660.
6. Singh D, Worst J, Singh R, Singh IR. Cataract and IOL. New Delhi: Jaypee Brothers Medical Publishers; 1995;163–165.
7. Nicholas AP. Brown Morphology of cataract and visual performance. Eye 1993;7:63–67.
8. Tulloh CG. Hereditary posterior polar cataract with report of a pedigree. Br J Ophthalmol 1955;39:374–379.
9. Nettleship E, Ogilvie FM. A peculiar form of hereditary congenital cataract. Trans Ophthalmol Soc UK 1996;26:19–20.
10. Primrose DA. A slowly progressive degenerative condition characterized by mental deficiency, wasting of limb musculature and home abnormalities, including ossification of the pinnae. J Ment Defic Res 1992;26:101–106.
11. Maumenee IH. Classification of hereditary cataracts in children by linkage analysis. Ophthalmology 1979;86:1554–1558.
12. Dark AJ, Streeten BW. Ultrastructural study of cataract in myotonia dystrophica. Am J Ophthalmol 1977;84:666.
13. Eshagian J, March WF, Goosens W, Rafferty MS. Ultrastructure of cataract in myotonic dystrophy. Invest Ophthal Vis Sci 1978;17:289.
14. Eshagian J, March WF, Goossens W. Ophthalmolog 1981;88:155.
15. Eshagian J. Human posterior subcapsular cataracts. Trans Ophthalmol Soc UK 1982;102:364–368.
16. Fine IH. Cortical cleaving hydrodissection. J Ref Surg 1992;18:508–512.
17. Vasavada AR, Desai JP. Stop, chop, chop & stuff. J Cataract Refract Surg 1996; 22(5):526–529.
18. Koch PS. Simplifying phacoemulsification. Thorofare, NJ: Slack Inc.; 1997;197–206.
19. Galand A. Consultation section. J Cat Ref Surg 1994; (20):99–104.
20. Gimbel HV, De Broff BM. Posterior capsulorrhexis with optic capture. Maintaining a clean visual axis after pediatric cataract surgery. J Cataract Refract Surg 1994;20:658–664.
21. Perkiness ES. Lens thickness in early cataract. Br J Ophthal 1988;72:348–353.

15

Phacoemulsification in Pediatric Patients

ALBERT W. BIGLAN

The management of cataracts in children is a more complex process than treating an adult patient who has previously developed presumably good visual acuity and has it diminished by opacification of the lens. In children, the visual system is in a process of development and will be incompletely developed until age 8 years. Amblyopia may be a determining factor in the final visual outcome in young children. The goal of cataract surgery in children is twofold: first, clear the visual axis to achieve the best possible visual acuity and secondly, to promote development of binocular visual function.

■ Anatomy of the Child's Eye

Children's eyes are different from adult eyes in several respects.[1,2] First, they are smaller; at birth the average axial length of the eye is 16.8 mm. The length will increase to the adult length of 23.6 mm by age 16. Most growth occurs during the first two years of childhood and by the end of the second year, the eye will have a mean axial length of 22 mm.

The second difference is the steepness of the corneal curvature. During development, the curvature of the cornea will change. At birth, very steep corneal topography readings are common, and will usually measure 47.00 to 51.00 D. The steep configuration decreases to adult readings of 43.50 D. A third consideration is the size of the lens. The horizontal diameter of the lens in an infant is 6.0 mm. This increases to 8.4 mm by 21 months and the lens diameter reaches an adult size, 9.3 mm, by 16 years.[3] The lens capsule in very young children does not lend itself to the current capsulorhexis techniques. It will tend to develop radially oriented tears. The lens substance in children is soft and the lens material or cataract is easily aspirated.

The child's eye has a more elastic sclera. Large incisions tend to make the eye collapse during surgery.

The vitreous is more viscous and formed and there may be a persistent attachment between the anterior hyaloid face and the posterior lens capsule. Remnants of the tunica vasculosa lentis may persist to some degree.

Frequently, developmental anomalies may coexist with a cataract. These defects may be ocular such as microphthalmia, foveal hypoplasia, optic nerve abnormalities, and persistence of the primary vitreous (PHPV) and of the tunica vasculosa lentis. Other defects will be systemic and include: heart, renal, or metabolic conditions which may cause cataracts and also increase risk for administration of general anesthesia. Cataract surgery in children is almost always performed under general anesthesia.

The visual system in children younger than 8 years is in a process of development. In adults, cataract surgery is associated with vision restoration. In children, the visual system is undergoing development and this needs to be facilitated. This proceeds rapidly during the first 3 or 4 months of life. The rate, and plasticity of development then progress at a slower rate up until the eighth year of life. During this period, amblyopia, deprivation, refractive, and strabismic, must be tested for and treated. Complications such as nystagmus, strabismus, or glaucoma may interfere with a good visual outcome.

There are other unique issues that are not experienced in the adult population. For example, children who have a cataract that involves only one eye, are going to be more difficult to achieve a high level of visual acuity because of the resistance of the child, and perhaps the parents, to occlude the good, normally functioning eye.

The onset of children's cataracts will vary. Cataracts may be congenital and present at birth or develop later during childhood. Often children have a propensity to develop a cataract as a result of a metabolic condition such as galactosemia. Other cataracts may be acquired following ocular trauma, radiation, inflammation or following administration of corticosteroids. Some partial cataracts will progress to complete lens opacities as is often the case with posterior lenticonus.

Successful management of cataracts in children requires a thorough understanding of the complex interplay between all of above issues. Additionally, the surgeon must have the facilities to provide safe general anesthesia for the child. If intraocular lens (IOL) rehabilitation is considered in a young or uncooperative child, equipment should be available in the operating room to perform keratometry and axial length measurements for lens power calculation.

■ Diagnosis of Cataracts in Children

Children almost never express symptoms related to cataracts. The ophthalmologist must rely upon signs to raise suspicion of the diagnosis. The parent may notice a whitish area in the pupil or the pediatrician may have difficulty examining the fundus during the newborn examination. When the cataracts involve both eyes and are complete, a very noticeable visual deprivation form of nystagmus will occur after 3 months of age. Once this low amplitude, low frequency form of pendular nystagmus ensues, attaining high levels of visual acuity (20/50 or better) is less likely.

Some lens defects may be present early in life (posterior lenticonus and PHPV) and the lens remains clear but may later develop opacification of the posterior lens capsule (Fig. 15–1). The same is true for metabolic

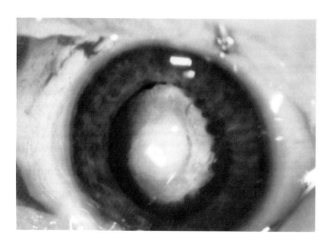

FIGURE 15–1. This eye has characteristic findings of P.H.P.V. Note the decreased horizontal corneal diameter (9.0 mm), the elongated ciliary processes and a very dense, thickened lens. An Ocutome combined with a Vannas scissors were needed to clear the visual axis.

conditions such as diabetes and galactosemia. Some early lens changes related to metabolic cataracts may be reversible with dietary alteration.

Inheritance

Cataracts may be inherited either as an autosomal dominant, autosomal recessive or with an X-linked pattern. Some genetically transmitted cataracts will occur as a result of inheriting a cataract producing metabolic or chromosomal disorder. Examination of other family members will help to clarify the inheritance pattern.

■ Classification of Cataracts

Cataracts may be classified by laterality, age of onset, extent, size-density, and by progression.[4-5]

Laterality

Cataracts can be classified as unilateral or bilateral. This classification is important because children with unilateral cataracts frequently have a delay in the detection of the cataract and for reasons already mentioned, the visual outcome may be less promising. Visual acuity in patients with bilateral congenital cataracts may be excellent if the cataracts are treated within the critical period of visual development or before the onset of nystagmus. In children with monocular cataracts, we have found this period to be before 17 weeks of age.[6]

Age of Onset

Cataracts may be described as congenital if they are present at birth or infantile if they are noticed in the perinatal period. Other cataracts may be acquired later in the child's life as a result of radiation, corticosteroid use, uveitis, or trauma. The term juvenile or adolescent are sometimes used to describe the cataract depending on the age the defect is noted.

The Extent and Location of Cataract

Partial cataracts may be capsular, zonular, cortical, nuclear or a combination of these. Cataracts may be pinpoint and involve only a small portion of the anterior lens capsule. These anterior polar cataracts will usually not show progression and a good visual outcome can be anticipated. Cataracts involving the posterior capsule will usually progress and have a greater impact in the measured visual acuity. Complete cataracts are those which obstruct the visual axis, even when viewed through a dilated pupil.

Some lenses may be clear but on retinoscopy will exhibit a double or distorted refracting system. Examples of these optical defects are seen with dislocated lenses, oil droplet cataracts, or posterior lenticonus or other defects in the posterior capsule of the lens. All of these share the same optical problem. They prevent a clearly focused form image from falling on the retina. When this occurs, development of visual acuity may be impeded and lens surgery should be considered.

Cataract Size and Density

The size of the cataract will have some influence on the level of visual acuity that is attainable. Opacities in the lens that are smaller than 2 mm can usually be observed with frequent monitoring of the vision. Cataracts 2.5 mm or larger will usually require surgery in order to clear the visual axis. Some partial opacities are flake or powder-like and others are opaque but small. Visual acuity may be surprisingly good in some children with partial cataracts. Lamellar cataracts may look "bad" but may not alter VA too much.

Progression

Cataracts may progress in their size or density with time or, in other unusual cases, cataracts may regress with dietary modification. Cataracts related to neonatal tetany and galactosemia may regress with correction of the metabolic defect through diet or medication. A transient haze may be present in the lens of premature infants during the early perinatal period. These "cataracts" will frequently regress without treatment.

Evaluation of the Child

Selected patients should be evaluated for cause of the cataract. The decision to proceed with an evaluation will be determined by the character of the cataract, its location, family history, type, and density of the opacity.[5-7] With this information and the findings on the physical examination to detect systemic problems, a focused laboratory investigation can be planned. A good cost-effective routine test is to examine the child's urine for reducing substances which will exclude galactosemia and diabetes. If the cataract has a lamellar character and is associated with neonatal tetany or infantile spasms, a serum calcium should be requested. A TORCH titer can exclude some common infectious causes for cataracts and is a test that is readily available in most laboratories. Patients with lens dislocation associated with Marfan syndrome or homocystinuria should have examinations focused on their cardiovascular system. Patients with Marfan syndrome have dilation of the aortic valve and other major vessels and patients with homocystinuria have an increase in coagulation which is treatable with vitamin B_6. If there is inflammation associated with cataract, studies should be ordered to rule out juvenile rheumatoid arthritis (JRA). Other tests that may be considered if the general physical exam includes suggestive findings are a serum and urine copper to exclude Wilson disease (sunflower cataract) and X-rays of the epiphyses of long bones to rule out Conradi syndrome.

Associated Ocular Defects

Associated defects should be investigated. Some of these defects will modify the procedure and instrumentation that will be used. Other defects may preclude cataract surgery. Eyes that have microphthalmia, as defined by a corneal diameter less than 9 mm, may not be good candidates for lens implantation. Microphthalmia may cause additional problems with instrumentation. Instruments designed for adult cataract surgery may be large and difficult to maneuver in small eyes. Eyes with extensive defects such as posterior staphylomas, optic nerve colobomas, and microphthalmia with cyst may not require cataract surgery because of the expected poor visual prognosis and the risk of loosing the eye as a result of surgery.

Nonsurgical Treatment

Not all pediatric cataracts require surgical treatment. Cataracts that are small and those which are partial and have areas where clear undistorted retinoscopy may require observation only. Frequent monitoring of the visual acuity by assessing the fixation response, watching for sensory strabismus, or measurement acuity using the Teller Visual Acuity Cards[R] are helpful for estimating acuity in nonverbal children. Caution must be exercised in interpreting the results because grating acuity will tend to underestimated amblyopia. As children mature, visual acuity may be quantitated using Allen cards, the Sheridan-Gardiner, E game, and with further maturation, Snellen letters.

■ Surgical Treatment

A visual acuity of 20/70 or less would suggest that cataract surgery is indicated. The decrease may be due to the cataract, amblyopia or a combination of these. The onset of strabismus or nystagmus related to visual deprivation is another indication for surgery. Some children who are very young or delayed developmentally may never subjectively provide a measured visual acuity. In these cases, the ophthalmologist's clinical judgment following assessment of the size, laterality of the cataract, will indicate if and when cataract surgery should be performed.

Congenital Cataracts

Children with a complete monocular congenital cataract should have surgery performed before 3 months of life.[6] Although there was emphasis at one time on operating and rehabilitating children immediately after birth,[8] it is now considered prudent to wait a week or two for the infant to become stable medically, to initiate diagnostic evaluations, and to have sufficient time to initiate appropriate pediatric and anesthesiology consultations to ensure the safety of the administration of general anesthesia.[9]

If cataracts involve both eyes, surgery should be performed on the eye with the denser opacity. Once this eye has recovered, (usually 2 to 3 weeks), cataract surgery should be performed on the fellow eye.

■ Optical Rehabilitation

Once a decision has been made to perform cataract surgery, the next consideration is selection of the method of optical rehabilitation that will be used. For patients with monocular cataracts, aphakic spectacles are not practical. Before 1 year of age, use of contact lens rehabilitation is suggested. After 1 year, an intraocular lens should be considered (Tables 15–1 and 15–2). In patients with bilateral cataracts, contact lens rehabilitation is recommended before 1 or 2 years. The unpredictable response and growth of an eye in a child younger than 1 year may preclude selection of an intraocular lens as a primary procedure in children.

Complete cataracts diagnosed at birth should be treated with cataract removal using a technique that preserves remnants of the anterior and posterior lens capsule leaflets. In

TABLE 15–1. Indications for Use of an IOL in Children

Unilateral Cataract
  Age 1–8 years old with a unilateral congenital cataract, expected or proven contact lens failure
  Age 1–17 years old with an acquired cataract with previously known adequate vision
  Unilateral developmental cataract age 1–17 years old
  Unilateral traumatic cataract
Bilateral Cataracts
  Patient older than 3 or 4 years of age
  Radiation induced cataracts
  Dry eyes
  Large amplitude nystagmus
  Eyelid scars

TABLE 15–2. Relative Contraindications for Pediatric IOL Implantation

Age less than 1 year
Microphthalmia
Microcornea (<9.0 mm cornea)
Glaucoma
Inflammation
Aniridia
Dislocated lens

most cases a primary posterior capsulotomy combined with an anterior vitrectomy should be performed. The eye should be rehabilitated with a contact lens. If the child becomes contact lens intolerant or when the child becomes mature, a secondary implant can be placed. Placement of an implant in a child younger than 1 year is technically difficult to perform and the response of a child's eye is unpredictable and in some situations, may be unfavorable to an implanted lens.

Infants who have bilateral complete, congenital cataracts should have cataract surgery performed and receive contact lens or spectacle rehabilitation. Once the eye becomes mature or the child becomes resistant to contact lenses or glasses, secondary implants can be considered.[10,11] Placement of an intraocular lens in a patient with bilateral acquired cataracts below the age of 2 to 4 years is considered by some authors to be unwise. This is due to our uncertainty about long-term effect and safety of implants as well as an incomplete understanding of the effect that an IOL has on the refractive error and growth of the eye over time. Children with a monocular cataract warrant the same concerns but the margin for safety and good vision is greater because of the presence of a sound fellow eye.

Socioeconomic Factors

The financial and social environment of the child's family may suggest one form of optical rehabilitation over another. Parents who are unable to insert and remove contact lenses are more likely to receive an IOL or spectacle correction if they have bilateral cataracts. Frequent loss of contact lenses may cause financial hardship.

■ The Cataract Procedure

Cataract surgery in children is almost exclusively performed under general anesthesia. It is necessary to have the pediatrician evaluate the cardiac and respiratory status before administering general anesthesia. In children under 1 year of age, cataract surgery is best accomplished in a hospital or short stay unit with appropriate back up medical services to access emergency care if needed.[9]

Obtaining blood samples from children for diagnostic evaluation may be psychologically traumatic. Blood samples for diagnostic purposes can be obtained at the time of the procedure. Once the child has an intravenous line established, blood samples may be obtained.

An adhesive urine collection bag can be given to the parents to collect a urine sample. Urine collected after a milk feeding should be tested with a Clinitest[R] strip to detect urine reducing substances. This test will screen for both diabetes and galactosemia. Other tests such as X-rays and genetic evaluations with karotyping should be performed in an out patient setting prior to the procedure.

Pupil Dilatation

Children younger than 6 months have their pupils dilated with 0.5% cyclopentolate (Cyclogyl[R]) and 2.5% phenylephrine (Neosynephrine[R]) drops applied twice, 5 minutes apart a half hour prior to coming to the operating room. Use of stronger concentrations of phenylephrine in children may cause elevated blood pressure and irritability of the myocardium. Older children will accept stronger concentrations of these mydriatic agents.

Patient Preparation

We routinely do not use prophylactic antibiotic or anti-inflammatory drops prior to surgery. The lashes are not trimmed. Once endotracheal anesthesia has been administered, axial length determinations can be performed using an A scan probe. If the lens is opaque, a B scan can also be performed. The corneal curvature is measured using one of several intraoperative keratometers such as the handheld Nidek-Marco (KM 500, Marco Ophth, Jacksonville, FL) or the Varidot[R] (Sysc Comp, Duncanville, TX) or a Terry keratometer[R]. If an IOL is going to be used, the pseudophakic lens power calculation can be made while the patient is being prepped.

Glaucoma is a problem that occurs in 25 to 31% of children who have a congenital cataract.[12–14] Presurgical and frequent postsurgical measurements of the intraocular pressure should be made with similar instrumentation so that valid comparison of the pressure can be made.

We use three instruments to document the intraocular pressure: the Perkins applanation tonometer, a Tonopen[R], and a Schiotz tonometer. There will frequently be small variations in the readings between these three instruments.

The patient's eye and surrounding area are prepped with a 5% Povidone-iodine (Betadine[R]) solution. The conjunctival cul-de-sacs are irrigated with a saline solution and at the completion of the prep, a drop of 5% Betadine[R] is instilled into the conjunctival cul-de-sac. An adhesive barrier drape is placed around the eye structures at this time. The lashes are retracted with the handle of a Weck-cel[R] sponge and an Opsite[R] adhesive cover is applied over the lashes to both cover and retract them.

The lids are separated using an open blade Kratz-Barraquer style lid speculum. For the past 15 years, I have not placed a superior rectus bridle suture because I like to be aware of the untethered position of the eye. When the eye begins to roll upward, this indicates that the level of anesthesia is light. Light anesthesia can be associated with increased tone of the extraocular muscles. If there is a large incision present, the risk of protrusion of eye contents increases.

Cataract Surgery, Without Placement of an Intraocular Lens

The selection of the incision site will be in some part modified by the training and experiences of the surgeon.

The pars plana or pars plicata incision offers the advantage of having increased ability to remove the lens and to perform an anterior vitrectomy through a single incision. However, there is a risk for hemorrhage, disinsertion of the ciliary body or the vitreous base, and to some degree there is some risk associated with blind passage of instruments behind the iris. Because of these potential problems, I prefer to use a limbal incision. I initially used a monoplane anterior limbal incision. Later I performed a three plane tunnel type of incision starting 2 mm back from the posterior limbus border. This scleral incision preserved the anterior chamber when the instruments were withdrawn but caused difficulty maneuvering instruments and made aspirating lens cortex at the 12 o'clock position. The advantage of a self-sealing, no stitch incision in a child is not a consideration since most surgeons will suture all wounds for safety. Children will often rub their eyes following surgery.

Over the past 3 years, I have again returned to the posterior-limbal region and performed a three plane incision at this site using a keratome. This incision provides direct observation of instruments as they are passed into the eye and is far enough anterior so that the lens cortex can be aspirated with greater ease. If an anterior vitrectomy is necessary, the suction-cutting probe can be used through the same incision.

A small peritomy or fornix based conjunctival flap is opened with a Vannas scissors. Entry is made into the anterior chamber using a 3.5 mm keratome using a three plane incision technique (Fig. 15–2). Viscoelastic is introduced into the anterior chamber with an attempt to make the lens-iris diaphragm bow posterior and become somewhat concave. Care should be exercised not to exaggerate this since an increase in the ocular pressure can occur and the vascular supply to the retina could be compromised. I have found that use of the visoelastic in the way described above will facilitate the anterior capsulorhexis. A needle with a bent tip is used to engage and tear the central portion of the anterior capsule. The flap of lens capsule is grasped with a Utrata or similar angled lens capsule forceps (Fig. 15–3). With frequent re-grasping of the flap and tearing toward the center of the lens while watching for radial tears, a continuous curvilinear capsulorhexis is attempted. This is a very difficult procedure to accomplish in patients younger than 4 years. If there is evidence of extension of the tear radially and it threatens to go to the equator of the lens, this procedure should be abandoned and the remainder of the capsule should be removed with a suction cutting device such as an Ocutome^R. The lens substance in children is soft and hydrodissection and hydrodelineation are not performed. The suction cutting device can be used in the aspiration mode, to remove the anterior lens cortex and the lens nucleus (Fig. 15–4). Ultrasound is rarely necessary. Once the nucleus has been aspirated, the peripheral lens cortex is removed from the fornices of the lens using either the Ocutome^R probe in a noncutting mode or preferably with a 0.3 mm I/A tip. It is best to have linear control of the suction pressure so that remnants of lens cortex can be engaged and then teased from the lens capsule without tearing the capsule. I find that 45 and 90 degree angled aspiration/irrigation probes greatly facilitate complete re-

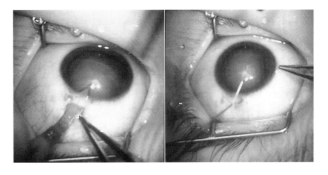

FIGURE 15–2. Left: After a peritomy has been made, a keratome is used to enter the anterior chamber creating a three plane incision. **Right:** The anterior chamber is deepened with a viscoelastic introduced through a cannula.

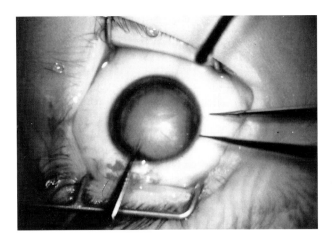

FIGURE 15–3. The tip of the Utrata capsulorhexis forceps is used to puncture the anterior lens capsule. Using a tearing motion with forces directed centrally, the anterior capsule is opened to a diameter of 5 mm. Care is taken to avoid tearing the capsule radially.

moval of lens cortex, especially at the 12 o'clock position (Fig. 15–4, Right). If the child is older than 5 or 6 years and will cooperate for a Nd:YAG laser capsulotomy, the posterior lens capsule, if it is clear, is left intact. However, if the child is too young or problems are anticipated with a Nd:YAG laser capsulotomy, a posterior capsulectomy and anterior vitrectomy should be performed using a suction cutting instrument. Attention to the size and location of the capsular opening is important. Care should be taken to make the anterior lens capsule opening slightly larger than the posterior lens capsule opening. The capsule leaflets will later fuse and form a baffle or a ring of support that may be important for stability of an IOL, if a secondary implant is required later. The pupil should be dilated frequently and kept moving to prevent iris-lens capsule adhesions from forming.

The anterior chamber is reestablished with balanced solution saline (BSS) and an iridectomy may be considered. If the child is at low risk for developing glaucoma or the iris is vascular, the surgeon may elect not to perform an iridotomy or an iridectomy. However, in patients with uveitis and in some patients with traumatic cataracts, performing an iridotomy or iridectomy may be prudent (Fig. 15–5). The incision may be self-sealing by design but it is safer to close all wounds in children with a 9–0 or 10–0 monofilament polygalactin 910 (vicryl[R]) suture. This will provide security if the child rubs the eye. Cephazolin (Kefzol[R]) 50 mg is injected subconjunctivally and dexamethasone (Decadron[R]), 4 mg/ml is injected into the Tenon's space at a separate site. The conjunctiva is replaced over the incision site and may be held in place by coaptation or a suture.

Postoperative care consists of drops and a shield. I prefer not to use a bandage dressing. Atropine 0.5% is used in children younger than 6 months of age and 1% atropine drops

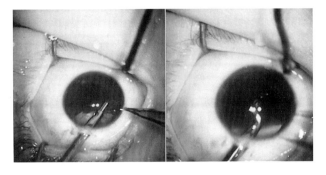

FIGURE 15–4. Left: The coaxial irrigating cannula of the Ocutome[R] tip is used to aspirate lens cortex. The cutting mode is used to complete the anterior capsulotomy and it can also be used to create an opening in the posterior capsule and remove the anterior hyaloid face. **Right:** A 45 degree angle aspiration-irrigation tip with a 0.3 mm opening is used to remove residual lens cortex in the 12 o'clock position. Cortex is grasped with the suction tip, moved centrally and the aspiration pressure is increased to aspirate the lens material.

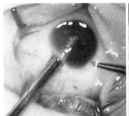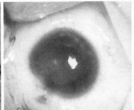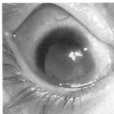

FIGURE 15–5. A variation of this technique is used to remove the cataract present in this eye with Peter's anomaly. **Left:** The anterior chamber is shallow, the cornea is small. In this patient the cornea had a horizontal diameter of 7.5 mm. **Center:** Following lensectomy and a central iridectomy or pupiloplasty, the red reflex is observed. **Right:** The eye 2 weeks later, demonstrating a good red reflex. The intraocular pressure was elevated slightly (24 mmHg).

are used twice a day in eyes of children older than 6 months. An antibiotic steroid combination such as Tobradex[R] may be used or Ocufloxacin[R] combined with a steroid such as Prednisolone acetate can be used during the postoperative period. The eye is shielded for 3 days and the patient is usually seen within 48 hours following surgery.

Topical medications are discontinued when inflammation has subsided. This is usually 2 or 3 weeks following surgery. Refraction is performed at this time and repeated frequently. Once the refraction is stable, contact lens or spectacle correction is prescribed.

In children who are younger than 2 years, bifocal is not added to the spectacle correction. Spectacles and contact lenses are set with a far point of 2/3 m. After age 2, patients who wear contact lenses receive overcorrection of spectacles which have a bifocal for near activities.

Cataract Surgery with Lens Implantation

Patient Selection

Patients with monocular cataracts who are older than 1 year or those who are contact lens resistant or those with inadequate family support to provide reliable and consistent application and removal of contact lenses are candidates for an IOL (Tables 15–1 and 15–2). The Federal Food and Drug Administration (FDA) has not approved IOL for use in children. Elaborate explanation and consent should outline the potential risks and benefits of this procedure. The parents should consent and if old enough, the child should assent to the procedure.

Lens Style and Power

The lens style should be biconvex and have a 6 to 6.5 mm optic diameter optic that has a UV coating. The haptics are angulated and should be between 12 and 13.5 mm in diameter with soft C or J loop configuration.

We and others have had recent favorable experience with use of the Acrysof[R] IOL.[15] The acrylic lens is able to be folded and inserted through a smaller incision. Additionally, this material is considered to produce reduced inflammation. We have used the 6 mm optic size for implantation in children. We choose this relatively large optic size because the lens capsule will frequently contract and displace the lens, even when the lens is within the capsular bag. The 6.0 mm optic provides a larger area of optical correction to provide an extra margin area if the lens is displaced within the capsular bag. Stager, et al. have been pleased with the performance of this lens in children.[15] Long-term studies regarding the safety and tolerance of pediatric eyes to this lens are lacking.

Lens Power

Measures should be taken to select a lens of appropriate power for the age of the child. Replacement of an IOL that has been placed in the eye of a child is difficult. Adhesions between the IOL and the lens capsule will be fibrotic and replacement or explanation of the lens will be difficult and hazardous. The power selection should be one that is appropriate for a lifetime. The surgeon should attempt to anticipate the refractive error at maturity. Some of the considerations in selecting a lens power are the age of the child, the refractive error of the fellow eye, and the refractive error of the parents. I calculate the lens power for the eye to achieve emmetropia using a SRK II formula.[16] Biometric readings may be difficult to obtain in children. If the child has not had axial length determination or is uncooperative for pre-operative studies, the axial length determination and keratometry are performed in the operating room after the child has been anesthetized. Lens power calculations are performed while the patient is being prepped and draped and the surgical microscope is being positioned.

There are a few studies that have evaluated the growth of the eye of primates and humans following cataract surgery with and without an IOL. The studies issue conflicting information on the growth patterns of the eye.[7,17-23] In children with dense lens opacities, the eye may have a longer than expected axial length. Other studies have shown that growth of the eye is reduced following implantation of a lens. Other studies have shown that the aphakic eye continues to elongate axially so that the correction of aphakia reduces with time even until age 20. We set as our goal to achieve a refractive error in adulthood that produces 1.50 D or less of anisometropia. In children younger than 2 years of age, the power selected should provide a final power that is close to the power that the fellow eye is expected to achieve. For example, if the fellow eye in a 2-year-old has a plano refractive error and the child has a traumatic cataract, it would be assumed that the power of the sound eye would eventually develop a myopic refractive error of about -2.00 D. If we calculated a lens power of +20.00 to achieve a plano refractive error in the injured eye, we would reduce the lens calculated power by -2.00 D and implant a +18.00 lens. Between 2 and 8 years of age, the lens power would be reduced by 1.50 D. In children older than 8 years of age, the refractive error is calculated to match the fellow eye.

Implantation of an Intraocular Lens

The technique used to implant an IOL is a modification of the procedure used to remove a cataract without an IOL. Style and power of the lens are selected and confirmed by the surgeon. If a difficult procedure is anticipated, intravenous mannitol may be given to contract the vitreous. This will facilitate maneuvering instruments in the anterior chamber. When mannitol is used, a dose of 200 mg/kg is administered intravenously by the anesthesia department as soon as the intravenous line has been established. When implanting a PMMA 6.5 mm optic lens, a fornix based conjunctival perimetry is made. A three plane incision is constructed at the mid-limbal position and entry is made into the anterior chamber with a keratome. Viscoelastic is introduced to partially fill the anterior chamber. A bent needle is used to puncture the anterior lens capsule and a capsulorhexis is performed with a Utrata capsulorhexis forceps. Hydrodissection is not performed. The lens material is removed as described in the previous section. After all cortical remnants are removed the posterior lens capsule is polished. If the posterior capsule is transparent, it is left intact. If there is a plaque or a dehiscence in the capsule, a posterior capsulectomy combined with a small anterior vitrectomy using the Ocutome[R] or similar suction cutting instrument is performed. We prefer the Ocutome[R] because it can be fit with a coaxial irrigating sleeve. If one desires, the sleeve can be removed and a separate irrigation cannula can be placed through a stab incision in the peripheral cornea. Viscoelastic is introduced into the anterior chamber. The limbal incision is increased to a cord length of 6.5 mm using corneal scissors. Viscoelastic is used to separate the lens capsule leaflets. The lens is irrigated with a balanced salt solution and the inferior haptic is inserted into the capsular bag under direct visualization (Fig. 15–6). The superior haptic is grasped with a nontooth forceps and, with gentle pressure, is inserted into the superior lens capsular bag. The lens is then dialed into position with a Sinsky hook so the lens is centered and the haptics are positioned with a 3 and 9 o'clock orientation. If the lens capsule has a radial tear that precludes lens placement within the capsular bag, the haptics may be alternatively placed in the ciliary sulcus. The haptics must both be either in the capsular bag or both in the ciliary sulcus. One in each position will cause decentra-

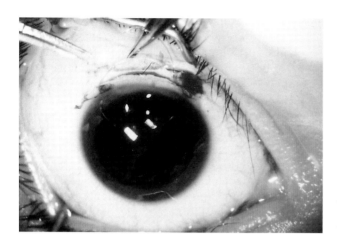

FIGURE 15–6. A 6.5 mm P.M.M.A. IOL is coated with viscoelastic and inserted through a 6.5 mm cord length incision. The haptics are placed in the capsular "bag" which has been opened with viscoelastic.

tion and possible iris capture. The corneal scleral wound is closed with four or five interrupted monofilament polygalactin 910 sutures. Two figures of eighth sutures may alternatively be used. Viscoelastic is aspirated from the anterior chamber. An iridotomy may be performed at this time. If the surgery has been uneventful and the patient is at low risk for developing glaucoma, an iridotomy or iridectomy is not performed.

When the posterior lens capsule is clear, we will leave it intact. We are fortunate to have access to the microruptor three Nd:YAG laser to treat capsular opacification (Fig. 15–7).[24] Alternative methods to "manage" the posterior capsule are to complete the lens implantation and then make a separate pars plana or a pars plicata incision with an MVR blade. An irrigation cannula is inserted into the anterior chamber and an Ocutome[R] or similar suction cutting device is placed through the pars plana incision to perform a posterior capsulotomy and removal of the anterior vitreous.[25]

Gimbel has described a capsulorhexis technique to open the posterior capsule. He performs this after he has implanted the lens.[26] The anterior capsule leaflet is reflected and a Utrata forceps is inserted behind the lens but above the surface of the posterior capsule to perform a posterior capsule capsulorhexis. A further modification that Gimbel has recently used is to prolapse the lens optic through the posterior capsule opening in effort to block lens epithelial cell migration in an effort to reduce the formation of secondary membranes.[27] These maneuvers are technically difficult to perform and there is an increased risk

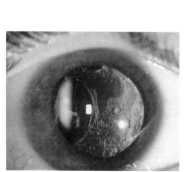
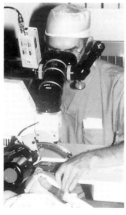

FIGURE 15–7. Left: A secondary membrane has caused the vision to decrease to 20/60. **Right:** A Nd:YAG laser is used to treat the membrane while the child is in the supine position under general anesthesia.

for creating a radial tear in the capsule which may cause the lens to decenter.

■ Secondary IOL Implantation in Children

Secondary IOL implantation in children is common because many children will have congenital complete cataracts that require removal at an age where implantation of a lens is not commonly performed.[10,11] When there is sufficient residual lens capsule to support a sulcus fixated IOL, fixation with a suture is not necessary. The technique for implanting a secondary IOL is similar for PMMA or the foldable lens. Viscoelastic is used to hydraulically separate the fused capsular leaflets from the iris. The cannula for the viscoelastic may be introduced through a peripheral iridotomy or iridectomy (Fig. 15–8). The firm adhesions between the iris and lens capsule can be separated with a Barraquer spatula. The cataract wound is extended with a corneal scissors and a 6.5 mm optic all PMMA lens is inserted. The haptics are placed in the ciliary sulcus. Alternatively, the wound can be enlarged with a 3.5 mm keratome and a foldable acrylic lens may be inserted into the ciliary sulcus (Fig. 15–9). The implants are dialed into position to be sure they are well centered and wound closure is similar for the other procedures.

Secondary Intraocular Lens Placement Without Capsular Support

In the previous decade, there was great concern about the formation of secondary membranes and their effect on treating amblyopia in children. Several surgeons advocated removal of the posterior lens capsule soon after the suction cutting instruments became available.[28] Some surgeons zealously removed the entire lens using a pars plana approach. When these children refuse to wear a contact lens or spectacles, placement of an IOL is difficult because of lack of capsular material to provide stabilization of an IOL.

Most surgeons feel uncomfortable about the placement of an anterior chamber IOL in a child. The long-term apposition of the lens haptic to the filtration angle and potential for loss of corneal endothelium and dislocation are valid concerns.[29,30] I have placed 14 secondary implants with suture fixation in children and young adults who have refused to wear contact lenses and have inadequate capsular support. This procedure is hazardous and the long-term outcome remains unclear. However, observing these implants over a period of 4 years, the eyes seem to tolerate the suture fixated implants well. The potential for endopthalmitis related to suture erosion is reduced by placing the 10-0 monofilament sutures that anchor the lens at the 3 and 9 o'clock position underneath a prepared half thickness scleral flap (Fig. 15–10). Lens tilt, dislocation, erosion of the suture or haptic and a risk for endopthalmitis are all valid concerns. However, suture placement is a reasonable alternative in these patients who are functionally aphakic.

■ Follow-Up Care

Following cataract surgery and optical rehabilitation with either contact lens or implant, am-

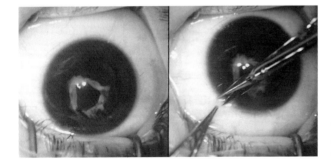

FIGURE 15–8. Left: The cataract was removed 2 years before. The capsule leaflets have fused and form a Sommering ring that will lend support for a secondary, sulcus fixated IOL. **Right:** A peritomy is created with a Vannas scissors.

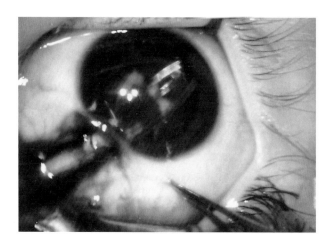

FIGURE 15–9. A 6.0 mm diameter foldable acrylic IOL is placed in the posterior chamber. The lens is stabilized between the iris and the capsule remnants. The haptics rest in the ciliary sulcus.

blyopia must be addressed. Overcorrection of the eye with spectacle lenses must be continuously updated to ensure that clear, focused images are placed on the retina during times when occlusion therapy is used. All children will opacify the posterior capsule. There is no way to prevent this.[31] The posterior capsule will opacify in approximately 2 to 3 years if the capsule is not opened at the initial surgical procedure.[31] Children who have had extensive posterior capsulotomies with anterior vitrectomies may still have sufficient growth of lens epithelium to require, in some cases, removal of secondary membranes using suction cutting instrument or a Nd:YAG laser. Repeat capsulotomies are common in children.

Following cataract surgery in children, it is common to require 15 to 25 office visits over the first year to monitor the clarity of the visual axis, the refractive error, and for those patients with contact lenses, to replace, adjust power, and fit of the contact. Later, the children need annual Follow-up visits to detect glaucoma, strabismus, and to continue to treat amblyopia.

■ Conclusion

Early identification and prompt surgical treatment of pediatric cataracts followed by prescription of accurate optical correction and amblyopia treatment will ensure the best visual result. Pre-existing eye conditions, absence of the fovea, undetected retinal problems, late onset glaucoma, secondary membrane formation, and difficulties in treatment of amblyopia are concerns to the treating ophthalmologist. Progress has been made in the management of children with cataracts. We

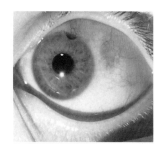 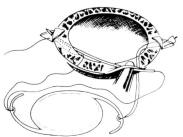

FIGURE 15–10. Left: When a child will not use a contact and monocular aphakic spectacles are rejected, a secondary IOL may be placed in the ciliary sulcus. If lens capsule is absent, the lens will require suture fixation. **Right:** This eye had a suture fixated PC IOL placed in the posterior chamber 3 months ago. The suture ends that secure the lens are protected by half thickness scleral flaps. These eyes should be followed for erosion of the conjunctiva and sclera over the suture. This can cause a risk for endophthalmitis.

must remember the progress that we have achieved in treating these children. Three decades ago, cataract surgery for children with unilateral complete cataracts was not a consideration. Results that are reported now frequently yield visual acuities better than 20/40 and in some patients, high levels of binocular function are being reported.

■ Tips and Pearls for Achieving the Optical Result When Managing a Child with a Cataract

1. Evaluate selected children for other disorders based on the character and location of the cataract.
2. Recognize that unilateral cataracts are going to be a greater challenge to achieve high levels of visual acuity.
3. Cataract surgery on eyes with complete cataracts should have the cataract removed and effective optical correction in place before 4 months of life.
4. The infant eye has an exuberant healing response following surgery and will tend to develop secondary membranes that are thick and will be difficult to open.
5. The child may not be cooperative and additional time must be expended to coax children to obtain a test or do an exam.
6. The parents must be recruited to be part of a team to rehabilitate the eye/eyes following surgery.
7. Children may require 20 to 30 visits during the first 2 years following surgery to maintain appropriate optical correction and treat amblyopia.
8. Refract, refract, refract. Prescribe frequently to maintain clear focused images on the fovea.
9. The corneal curvature, axial length of this eye will change rapidly during the first 2 years of life making selection of an IOL with a correct power difficult.
10. Children with cataracts will have amblyopia (>50%), glaucoma (30%), strabismus (>50%) and secondary membranes (100%), that will require early detection and effective treatment to ensure an optimal result.
11. Failure to treat coexisting amblyopia will negate the best surgical result.

REFERENCES

1. Gordon RA, Donzis PB. Refractive development of the human eye. Arch Ophthalmol 1985;103:785–789.
2. Inagaki Y. The rapid change of corneal curvature in the neonatal period and infancy. Arch Opthalmol 1986;104:1026–1027.
3. Bluestein EC, Wilson ME, Wang X-H, Rust PF, Apple DJ. Dimensions of the pediatric crystalline lens: implications for intraocular lenses in children. J Pediatr Ophthalmol Strabismus 1996;33:18–20.
4. Biglan AW, Cheng KP. Pediatric cataracts and systemic diseases current concepts in ophthalmology. Pennsylvania Medicine 1994;(suppl):35–41.
5. Biglan AW, Cheng KP. Cataracts in infants and children. In: Margo CE, Hamed LM, Mames RN (eds). Diagnostic problems in clinical ophthalmology. Philadelphia: WB Saunders; 1994;802–810.
6. Cheng KP, Hiles DA, Biglan AW, Pettapiece MC. Visual results after early surgical treatment of unilateral congenital cataracts. Ophthalmology 1991;98:903–910.
7. Lambert SR, Drack AV. Infantile cataracts. Surv Ophthalmol 1996;40:427–458.
8. Beller R, Hoyt CS, Marg E, Odom JV. Good visual function after neonatal surgery for congenital monocular cataracts. Am J Ophthalmol 1981;91:559–565.
9. Woelfel SK, Brandon BW. Anesthesia for the pediatric ophthalmology patient. In: Tasman W, Jaeger EA (eds). Duane's Clinical Ophthalmology. Philadelphia: Lippincott Raven; 1995;1–17.
10. Devaro JM, Buckley EG, Awner S, Seaber J. Secondary posterior chamber intraocular lens implantation in pediatric patients Am J Ophthalmol 1997;123:24–30.
11. Biglan AW, Cheng KP, Davis JS, Gerontis CC. Secondary intraocular lens implantation after cataract surgery in children. Am J Ophthalmol 1997;123:224–234.
12. Simon JW, Mehta N, Simmons ST, et al. Glaucoma after pediatric lensectomy/vitrectomy. Ophthalmology 1991;98:670–674.
13. Mills MD, Robb RM. Glaucoma following childhood cataract surgery. J Pediatr Ophthalmol Strabismus 1994;31:355–360.
14. Johnson CP, Keech RV. Prevalence of glaucoma after surgery for PHPV and infantile cataracts. J Pediatr Ophthalmol Strabismus 1996;33:14–17.
15. Stager DR, Jr, Stager DR, Sr, Wilson ME, et al. Foldable acrylic intraocular lenses in children presented at the 23rd Annual Meeting of the American Association for Pediatric Ophthalmology and Strabismus. Charlestown, SC. April 1997.

16. Sanders DR, Retzlaff J, Kraff M. Comparison of the SRK II formula and other second generation formulas. J Cataract Refract Surg 1988;14:136–141.
17. Raviola E, Wiesel TN. An animal model of myopia. N Engl J Med 1985;312:609–615.
18. Von Noorden GK, Lewis RA. Ocular axial length in unilateral congenital cataracts and blepharoptosis. Invest Ophth Vis Sci 1987;4:750–752.
19. Fernandes A. Aphakia, pseudophakia and occlusion: effects on postnatal axial eye elongation in a monkey model. In Cotlier E, Taylor D, Lambert S (eds). Congenital Cataracts. London: Landes Co.; 1994;189–199.
20. Rasolly R, Ben Ezra D. Congenital and traumatic cataract. The effect on ocular axial length. Arch Ophthalmol 1988;106:1066–1068.
21. Moore BD. Changes in the aphakic refraction of children with unilateral congenital cataracts. J Pediatr Ophthalmol Strabismus 1989;26:290–295.
22. Sinsky RM, Stoppel JO, Amin PA. Ocular axial length changes in a pediatric patient with aphakia and pseudophakia. J Cataract Refract Surg 1993;19:787–788.
23. Kora Y, Inatomi M, Fukado Y, Marumori M, Yaguchi S. Long-term study of children with implanted intraocular lenses. J Cataract Refract Surg 1992;18:485–488.
24. Atkinson CS, Hiles DA. Treatment of secondary posterior capsular membranes with the Nd:YAG laser in a pediatric population. Am J Ophthalmol 1994;118:496–501.
25. Buckley EG, Klombers LA, Seaber JH, Scalise-Gordy A, Minzter R. Management of the posterior capsule during pediatric intraocular lens implantation. Am J Ophthalmol 1993;115:722–728.
26. Gimbel HV, Ferensowicz M, Raanan M, DeLuca M. Implantation in children. J Pediatr Ophthalmol Strabismus 1993;30:69–79.
27. Parks MM. Posterior lens capsulectomy during primary cataract surgery in children. Ophthalmology 1983;90:344–345.
28. Gimbel HV. Posterior capsulorhexis with optic capture in pediatric cataract and intraocular lens surgery. Ophthalmology 103:1871–1875.
29. Sharpe M, Biglan AW, Gerontis CG. Scleral fixation of posterior chamber lenses in children. A case series. Ophthal Surg Lasers 1996:27:325–330.
30. Dahan E, Sahmenson BD, Levin J. Ciliary sulcus reconstruction for posterior implantation in the absence of an intact posterior capsule. Ophthalmic Surg 1989;20:776–780.
31. Plager DA, Lipsky SN, Snyder SK, et al. Capsular management and refractive error in pediatric intraocular lenses. Ophthalmology 1997;104:600–607.

16

Phacoemulsification Following Vitreoretinal Surgery

LOUIS D. NICHAMIN

As the indications for vitrectomy surgery accrue, there follows a growing population of cataract patients who, in their vitrectomized state, will challenge the phaco surgeon. These patients require special consideration because of their altered physiologic state as well as for the underlying pathology which necessitated the vitreoretinal procedure. Nonetheless, with careful planning and subtle but important modifications in surgical technique, the vast majority of these patients may enjoy the myriad benefits of modern small-incision phaco surgery.

■ Preoperative Considerations

As with any special circumstance, the time spent prior to surgery formulating a specific plan will in the end prove to be a prudent investment. As concentration is focused upon refinements for the most effective phaco procedure, the cataract surgeon must remain cognizant of the patient's entire state of ocular health. Circumspect decision-making, as for example in intraocular lens (IOL) selection, is needed in order to afford the patient the greatest overall benefit.[1]

History

Not only must the nature of the vitreoretinal pathology be known, but the extent of the previous surgery should be understood since it will bear directly upon the success or complexity of the phaco procedure. An eye having had a limited core vitrectomy for removal of an epiretinal membrane will behave differently than an eye that has undergone extensive vitreous dissection for a complicated retinal detachment. Lengthy surgery, multiple procedures, and anterior vitreous dissection all predispose to a higher likelihood of compromised zonules and possible capsular defects.

Most vitrectomized eyes, particularly in diabetics, are unusually prone to developing clinically significant cystoid macular edema. Pre- and postoperative treatment with topical nonsteroidal anti-inflammatory medications may help to reduce this problem.[2] Diabetic patients should have existing retinopathy controlled preoperatively, and should be made aware that their retinopathy may worsen despite uncomplicated surgery.[3,4]

Following extensive vitreous surgery, particularly in young myopic patients, scleral rigidity will be unusually low and additional support by way of a Flieringa ring or a separate (self-maintaining) infusion source may prove useful.

Examination

The preoperative exam should make note of several important findings. Conjunctival and limbal scarring may influence incision location, as opposed to routine cases where astigmatic concerns dominate. The combination of a prominent brow, a deeply set eye and an unusually deep anterior chamber, as is commonly encountered following vitrectomy, all make for compounded difficulty during surgery. Thus, a temporal approach is generally preferred. Increased episcleral scarring and bleeding should be anticipated in the vicinity of the previous entry ports, typically located 3.5 mm posterior to the limbus at the superonasal, superotemporal, and inferotemporal locations. The choice of IOL (as discussed below) will also influence the incision design.

A compromised corneal endothelium may be present if multiple procedures have been performed, particularly if silicone oil was in place for a significant length of time. Pupillary dilation may be limited secondary to underlying disease or previous surgical manipulation. Vigorous dilating agents should be used, and preoperative use of a topical nonsteroidal anti-inflammatory may help reduce intraoperative miosis which occurs more frequently in these eyes. One must be prepared to employ one of the multiple techniques that now exist for effective pupillary enlargement.[5]

During biomicroscopy, subtle irido or phacodonesis should be sought for since some of these cases will have compromised zonules. If seen, careful gonioscopy should be performed to better delineate the extent of the weakened zonules. A number of specific technique modifications exist for this condition[6,7]; incision placement opposite to the dialysis, modified capsulorhexis and phaco techniques, and use of an endocapsular ring (see below) should all be considered.[8]

The Surgical Plan

An important issue that needs to be considered preoperatively is the form of anesthesia to be used. Increasingly, phaco surgeons are learning of the benefits of noninjection anesthesia.[9] One of the very few times when topical anesthesia may not provide adequate patient comfort is during maneuvers that stretch the zonular network. As in high myopes, the vitrectomized eye will experience an increase in zonular stretch and lens/iris diaphragm movement. This undesirable sensation may be eliminated through the use of intracameral nonpreserved lidocaine, but enhanced posterior diffusion of the anesthetic in the vitrectomized eye may lead to a temporary retinal blockade and attenuation of visual function.[10] Although electrophysiologic studies have not been performed following this phenomenon, visual recovery has always been complete with no recognizable sequelae. For similar reasons, other additives to the infusion bottle should be carefully considered, and aminoglycoside antibiotics should likely be avoided.

Alternatively, conventional injection anesthesia may be used. The increased orbital volume may, in fact, help to negate the diminutive vitreous pressure present following a vitrectomy and reduce the overly deep anterior chamber depth. For the same reason, oculopressive devices and massage should be avoided. In addition, injection anesthesia will better permit a subconjunctival anti-inflammatory injection at the conclusion of surgery if desired.

Another very important preoperative decision involves the choice of an IOL. Both the biomaterial used and the lens design itself will affect the long-term health, stability, and future disease management of the patient's eye. Two issues in particular must be considered. First, one must expect an increased tendency toward breakdown of the blood aqueous barrier and therefore higher levels of inflammation. Evidence is accumulating to suggest that the more hydrophilic biomaterials are better suited in these circumstances, as are surface-treated IOL's.[11] The second consideration revolves around the ability to maintain maximal visualization through the implant. Silicone implants may not be ideal if the patient is likely to undergo an air/fluid exchange[12] or require a vitreous substitute such as silicone oil.[13] Visualization may also be hampered by lens designs utilizing small optics, ovoid optics, small capsulorhexis diameters, and inadequate capsular polishing.[14,15] Given the possibility that capsular or zonular defects may be present and that future surgical manipulation may be required, fixation stability is also an important concern. Current one-piece plate haptic IOL designs are not optimal in this setting. Newer three-piece foldable IOLs with PMMA or polyimide haptics yield good fixation qualities; however, rigid one-piece all PMMA designs probably provide the best long-term stability.[16]

A final note regarding IOL selection relates to lens power calculation. Many of these eyes are naturally myopic, or increased axial length may have been induced by an encircling scleral buckle. Third generation formulae should be used for optimal results. One must also be aware that the refractive index of silicone oil makes it behave as though it were an "intraocular minus lens." Therefore, without an appropriate power adjustment, significant hyperopic overcorrections would be expected. Hoffer suggested that the standard ultrasound velocity of 1555 M/sec be adjusted to 1000 M/sec in these eyes.[17] Even with this adjustment, biometry may prove difficult with false retinal spikes encountered and therefore a tendency toward hyperopic overcorrections. It has further been suggested that convex-plano-shaped IOLs (with the plano surface positioned posteriorly) be used to minimize this problem.[18] It should be kept in mind that a myopic shift will occur once the silicone oil is removed. If a "refractive surprise" does result, secondary, piggy-back IOLs may prove useful as opposed to IOL removal and/or exchange.

■ Intraoperative Considerations

Prior to initiating the phaco incision, the globe should be firmed up by performing an aqueous-viscoelastic exchange through a side-port incision. Vitrectomized eyes tend to be soft and therefore encourage a more shallow tunnel dissection. This tendency is further promoted if episcleral tissue is not cleanly dissected prior to performing a scleral tunnel incision. Both the phaco and side-port incisions should be carefully crafted to avoid unnecessary fluid leakage since fluid dynamics become increasingly important in these eyes.

When performing the capsulorhexis, avoid overfilling the anterior chamber with viscoelastic since these chambers, as noted, are unusually deep. A large (5.5 to 6.0 mm) capsulorhexis will facilitate lens removal and help prevent peripheral capsular opacification and possible capsular phimosis secondary to weakened zonules. Controlling a larger rhexis is aided by working through the smallest possible internal incision opening, which will prevent loss of the viscoelastic, shallowing, and excursion of the tear out to the periphery. This, however, should be a rare circumstance given the unusually deep anterior chamber that is so commonly encountered in this scenario.

Gentle but very thorough hydrodissection is then performed. Be aware that a capsular defect may be present posteriorly and slow, gentle hydrodissection followed by frequent decompression will help avoid a "blowout." Adequate lens rotation should be verified prior to phaco to assure that unnecessary capsular and zonular stress do not occur.

Because of increased lens/iris diaphragm movement in these eyes, fluidics become extremely important. Bottle height should be lowered since anterior chamber depth will be greater than usual. It should also be noted that these patients are more prone to the infusion deviation syndrome wherein fluid migrates posteriorly through the zonular network, increases the volume of the vitreous compartment, and thereby creates shallowing of the anterior chamber. Raising the infusion bottle only worsens this paradoxical problem.

■ Phaco Technique

Regarding phaco technique, the approach depends upon individual surgeon preference and experience. In the face of very loose zonules, a nonrotational technique such as Fine's chip-and-flip or Gimbel's phaco sweep may prove useful. In addition, a large capsulorhexis followed by hydro and viscodissection may allow manipulation of the lens out of the loose capsular bag for safer removal.

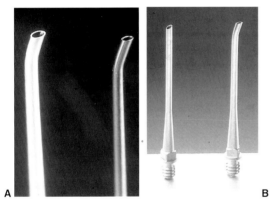

FIGURE 16–1 (A, B). Angled Kelman phaco needle, Alcon Labs, Fort Worth, Texas.

When sculpting or grooving, access to the lens and hence "angle of attack" may be more efficient if an angled (at the hub) Kelman phaco needle is used (Fig. 16–1). Furthermore, sufficient phaco power and a more highly beveled needle tip will help prevent pushing and chattering of the lens, and therefore diminish zonular stress. The lens manipulator may also provide countertraction to stabilize the nucleus during this stage. Employing hydrodelineation to define an outer epinuclear shell affords the surgeon additional safety while performing endocapsular manipulations.

Chopping and cracking maneuvers should be performed slowly and carefully. The higher vacuum and flow settings currently used to evacuate disassembled lens fragments should not be too extreme given the likelihood of capsular and zonular tenuity. If zonular integrity is poor, an endocapsular ring may be placed prior to epinucleus and cortex removal in order to avoid capsular bag collapse. Cortical cleanup should be performed with lower I & A settings for similar reasons. Circumferential stripping reduces direct radial traction on the zonules. In extreme cases, a manual technique should be used for the greatest safety. Thorough removal of residual lens epithelial cells is desirable to decrease the need for subsequent YAG laser intervention and thereby minimize further retinal complications; however, polishing maneuvers must be performed very gently to avoid disinsertion of zonules.

■ Lens Implantation

As stated, the selection of an IOL must take into account long-term fixation and stability concerns as well as optimize visualization of the posterior segment. Regardless of lens style, placement must be performed gently, minimizing rotational maneuvers. If an area of distinct zonular weakness exists, one haptic should be placed directly into this location to extend the capsular fornix. Alternatively, an endocapsular ring may be used in conjunction with the intraocular lens. This ring, (Morcher, Stuttgart, Germany) is made of PMMA and comes in two sizes, 10 mm for normal axial lengths and 12 mm for unusually large eyes (Fig. 16–2). This ring acts to evenly distend and fixate the equatorial portion of the capsular bag. US surgeons must be aware that FDA approval of this device is pending, and appropriate informed consent and possibly investigational review board approval may need to be obtained.

Upon completing the case, care must be taken to avoid sudden hypotony, such as when removing the viscoelastic. This increases instability of the posterior segment and might permit prolapse of residual vitreous. Instruments

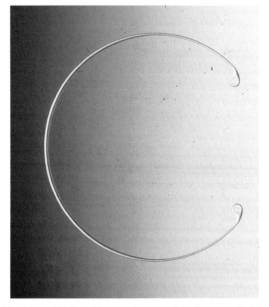

FIGURE 16–2. The endocapsular ring, available from Morcher, Stuttgart, Germany.

should be slowly removed from the phaco incision as the anterior chamber is reconstituted through the side-port incision. Of course, a watertight closure must be confirmed; altered scleral rigidity and perilimbal scarring may necessitate placement of sutures.

■ Postoperative Considerations

As previously mentioned, these patients are more inclined toward developing cystoid macular edema and therefore should be treated vigorously with anti-inflammatory medications postoperatively. Subconjunctival injections, although often omitted today after routine surgery, should be considered. Frequent topical corticosteroids may be supplemented with topical nonsteroidal anti-inflammatory medications and a more gradual taper is recommended. On occasion, fibrin accumulation may occur which may be successfully managed through the use of intracameral tissue plasminogen activator.[19] Cycloplegic agents should not be overlooked.

Even if the patient's underlying vitreoretinal pathology was mild in nature and the phaco procedure uncomplicated, a rigorous evaluation of the peripheral fundus is warranted. Patients should be counseled to immediately report new photopic phenomena.

■ Conclusion

By recognizing the differences in the physiologic state of the vitrectomized eye, and keeping in mind the nature of the patient's previous vitreoretinal pathology, today's cataract surgeon may readily adapt modern small incisional phaco technique to this challenging patient population. The principles discussed will hopefully minimize surgical difficulty and help reduce complications.

■ Tips and Pearls

1. Liberal use of steroid and nonsteroidal topical medications, both pre- and postoperatively.
2. Expect poor pupillary dilation and employ pupilloplasty techniques.
3. Search for irido or lenticulodonesis preoperatively.
4. Expect to encounter weakened zonules or occult capsular defects intraoperatively.
5. Avoid massage or softening measures prior to surgery.
6. Firm up IOP prior to incision.
7. Careful IOL selection; maximize biocompatibility, fixation stability, and postoperative visualization.
8. Avoid excessive deepening of anterior chamber by lowering bottle height.
9. Perform thorough hydrodissection.
10. Minimize endocapsular rotational maneuvers.
11. Lower vacuum or use manual techniques for cortical cleanup.

REFERENCES

1. Nichamin LD. New IOL choices have implications for patients with retinal disorders. Ocular Surg News 1992;10(9):69.
2. Miyake K. The significance of inflammatory reactions following cataract extraction and intraocular lens implantation. J Cataract Refract Surg 1996;22(Suppl.): 759–868.
3. Dowler JGF, Hykin PG, Lightman SL, Hamilton AM. Visual acuity following extracapsular cataract extraction in diabetics: a meta-analysis. Eye 1995;9:313–317.
4. Cunliffe IA, Flanagan DW, George NDL, Aggarwaal RJ, Moore AT. Extracapsular cataract surgery with lens implantation in diabetics with and without proliferative retinopathy. Br J Ophthalmol 1991;75:9–12.
5. Nichamin LD. Enlarging the pupil for cataract extraction using flexible nylon iris retractors. J Cataract Refract Surg 1993;19:793–796.
6. Nichamin LD. Zonular dialysis: reducing the "stress." Presentation at 5th Annual Ocular Surgery News Symposium, New York City, NY, October 5, 1996.
7. Nichamin LD. Zonular dialysis: reducing the "stress." Award-winning video, ASCRS Film Festival April 30, 1997.
8. Witschel B, Legler UFC. The capsular ring. Cionni RJ. Clinical Experience in the U.S.A. Video Journal of Cataract and Refractive Surgery. 1993;9(4).
9. Dillman DM. Topical anesthesia for phacoemulsification. Ophthalmol Clin North Am, 1995;8(9):419–427.
10. Nichamin LD. Letter to the editor. Ocular Surg News, 1997;15(4):8.
11. Apple DJ. Silicone IOLs not indicated in every patient. Ocular Surg News 1996;14:22.
12. Hainsworth DP, Chen SN, Cox TA, Jaffe GJ. Conden-

sation on polymethyl methacrylate, acrylic polymer, and silicone intraocular lenses after fluid-air exchange in rabbits. Ophthalmology 1996;103:1410–1418.
13. Apple DJ, Federman JL, Krolicki TJ, et al. Irreversible silicone oil adhesion to silicone intraocular lenses. Ophthalmology 1996;103:1555–1562.
14. Masket S, Geraghty BS, Crandall AS, et al. Undesired light images associated with ovoid intraocular lenses. J Cataract Refract Surg 1993;19:690–694.
15. Masket S. Postoperative complications of capsulorhexis. J Cataract Refract Surg 1993;19:721–724.
16. Apple DJ, Solomon KD, Tetz MR, et al. Posterior capsule opacification—major review. Surv Ophthalmol 1992;37:73–116.
17. Hoffer KJ. Ultrasound velocities for axial length measurement. J Cataract Refract Surg 1994;20(9):554–562.
18. Holladay JT. Modern Implant Surgery XVI: Clear Corneal Phaco. Presented at American Academy of Ophthalmology Meeting. Chicago, IL, October 30, 1996.
19. Lesser GR, Osher RH, Whipple D, et al. Treatment of anterior chamber fibrin following cataract surgery with tissue plasminogen activator. J Cataract Refract Surg 1993;19:301–305.

17

Phacoemulsification in Ocular Trauma

MIGUEL ÂNGELO PADILHA

When handling a traumatic cataract, important considerations should be taken into account when such cases are being examined.

The level of involvement of the anterior segment will guide the surgical course to be taken in each case. Among possible complications are a minor or extensive corneal laceration, at times accompanied by an scleral rupture, the possible presence of an iris incarceration, iridodialysis, hyphema, vitreous in the anterior chamber, lens subluxation, displacement of the lens into the anterior or posterior chamber (or even into the vitreous).

The causal agent of the trauma, the level of inflammatory reaction present, the availability of appropriate material for the surgical repair, as the familiarity of the surgeon in handling the anatomical elements of the anterior and posterior segment, and the implantation of scleral-fixated intraocular lenses, should be duly assessed prior to surgery.

In those cases where a traumatic cataract is a result of a perforation, the surgeon should remember the possible compromise of the posterior capsule during its extraction.

Another important consideration in the handling of these cases is related to whether the patient should be subjected to local or general anesthesia. As a general rule, when there is an extensive corneal or corneo-scleral laceration, shallowing of the anterior chamber and ocular hypotension, it seems more appropriate to use general anesthesia while local anesthesia is considered in cases where damage is considered minimal.

■ Diagnosis and Conduct

A number of traumatic etiologies may lead to lens opacification. In those caused by a high-voltage electric shock or after being struck by lightening, the lens opacification frequently bilateral, may take place over a period of minutes through a few days. In general, this type of cataract is posterior subcapsular (Figs. 17–1A and B) or have a white, milky appearance over the entire lens due to precipitation of proteins (Fig. 17–2).

The procedure in these cases is the same as for standard phacoemulsification with in-the-bag implantation of an artificial lens. The chief surgical difficulty is during capsulorhexis with a total cataract. Turning the operating room lights off to improve contrast and increasing the light from the surgical microscope under high magnification may facilitate this surgical step. Should the continuous

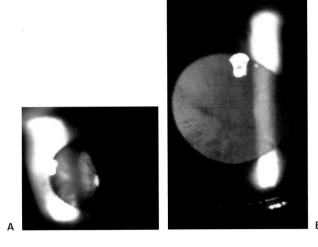

FIGURE 17–1. **(A,B)** Galvanic cataract (posterior subcapsular).

curvilinear capsulotomy nevertheless prove unfeasible, handle the surgery with the more traditional "can-opener" technique (Fig. 17-3 and 17-4).

In cases of direct contusion to the eyeball or head concussion, a subluxation or luxation of the lens may occur. As an example of the latter, we will mention cases of direct ocular trauma caused by a tennis ball where a complete zonular rupture allows the lens to fall entirely into the vitreous body.

In this type of accident, treatment may be conservative provided that the lens is almost immobile in the inferior section of the eyeball. Should it be totally loose within the vitreous, the possibility of causing retinal detachment is considered high, thus requiring its prompt removal. A retinal surgeon will be more familiar handling this type of complication through a lensectomy, vitrectomy, and fixation of an intraocular lens (IOL) to the sclera.

Under other circumstances, displacement of the lens into the anterior chamber may take place. In these cases, the presence of vitreous in the anterior chamber is almost always noticed as well as an increased intraocular pressure. When anterior lens luxation is present and/or glaucoma secondary to a pupillary block, surgery should be performed immediately.

We believe that the most appropriate procedure in this situation is the intracapsular lensectomy followed by implantation of a Kelman-type anterior chamber intraocular lens.

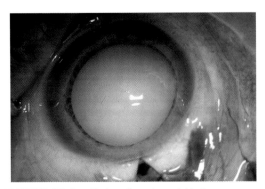

FIGURE 17–2. Galvanic cataract (left eye; same patient as in Figure 1).

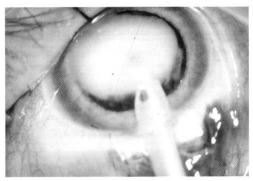

FIGURE 17–3. Phacoemulsification in soft cataract (galvanic cataract).

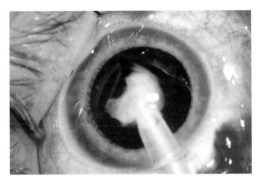

FIGURE 17–4. Final stage of phacoemulsification. No residual cortical material is present.

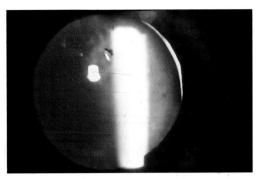

FIGURE 17–5. Zonular dyalisis is present between 1 and 3 o'clock.

Almost always, an ample anterior vitrectomy is necessary prior to lens implantation. In the case of a relatively young patient or when the conditions of the corneal endothelium are not favorable for this type of lens, a scleral-fixated posterior chamber intraocular lens implantation should be performed.

In cases of a lens luxation into the posterior chamber itself, the patient may complain of monocular diplopia. Depending on the symptoms present, a contact lens may be adapted. If an increase in the intraocular pressure occurs, it can be easily controlled. The surgery may be posponed, and should be performed as in the previously described situation.

In some cases of subluxation, the zonular rupture might be very small. At times it might even be difficult to detect a zonular rupture, requiring an ample mydriasis to make the correct diagnosis (Fig. 17–5). Iridodonesis may be observed. Slit lamp examination will demonstrate the difference in distances between the pupillary border and the anterior lens capsule at various points (Figs. 17–6A and B). Opacification of the lens often occurs at an early stage.

Under ample mydriasis, we can better evaluate the condition and choose the appropriate surgical technique. In presence of a small zonular rupture involving less than 45 degrees of the entire zonular ring, phacoemulsification may be performed in the standard manner. In such cases, a good hydrodissection must be obtained. This is of vital importance to prevent extension of the zonular dialysis at the time of the phacoemulsification and aspiration of the lens cortical material. There is controversy with regard to whether or not it is necessary to use the PMMA endocapsular rings to hold and distend the capsular bag. We feel that implantation of the endocapsular rings might not be essential in most cases, given the fact that when a very extensive zonular dialysis is present, the risk of displacing the entire bag, including the implanted IOL, is possible even in presence of such rings. You may consider using the ring to add support to a sulcus-fixated IOL.[1]

Should the zonular rupture be equal or greater than 180 degrees (Fig. 17–7), it is very likely that vitreous will be present during the surgery. We believe that the intracapsular technique is the most appropriate in these situations, followed by the implantation of an anterior chamber IOL or a sutured posterior chamber lens to the scleral wall.

In perforating traumas, it is not only the cornea or sclera that may be involved, but the iris, the ciliary body, the lens, the retina, and the vitreous. When the lens is injured, opacification is almost always immediate. Depending on the causative agent and the site of penetration, this opacity may be limited to a small area, particularly when the iris is also affected. The inflammatory reaction induced will add to healing of the anterior capsule. When the opacification is minimal, not progressive and off-axis, there will be no indication for surgery.

Should the injury be more extensive including rupture of the anterior capsule, surgery is

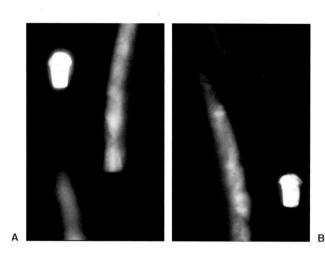

FIGURE 17–6. **(A)** Slit lamp shows a space between the iris and the lower part of the anterior capsule of the lens. **(B)** At the upper part, almost no space is present.

then indicated and, in this case phacoemulsification is almost always limited to aspiration of the cortical matter present.

However, much care should be taken when there is evidence of scleral laceration or a corneal perforation. In accidents involving broken vehicle windshields, small glass fragments may penetrate the cornea without a clearly visible wound. It will be only at the time of the cataract surgery that the presence of these intra-lenticular foreign bodies will be detected.[2]

When there is a metallic foreign body present in the vitreous or in contact with the retina, much care should be taken with the use of electromagnets. It is possible to cause greater intraocular trauma when extracting the fragment. If at all possible, forceps should be used for this type of removal.

After antibiotics and steroidal and nonsteroidal anti-inflammatory drug for 24 hours, surgery should be performed under appropriate anesthesia. Phacoemulsification should be performed carefully, taking into account the probable rupture of the posterior capsule. Aspiration of the lens material is almost always sufficient. If a ruptured posterior capsule is found, the BSS infusion should be lowered to reduce anterior chamber turbulence and expansion of the capsular rupture. Then, under the constant presence of a viscoelastic material, aspiration of cortical remnants is performed using a two-way cannula, or a cannula mounted on a 3 cc syringe (the dry aspiration) as suggested by Stegman.[3]

If possible, a posterior capsulorhexis of the posterior capsule should be attempted with the Utrata or the long Kelman-McPherson forceps.

The selection of the IOL to be implanted will depend on the extent of the posterior capsule rupture. If small, an IOL 12 mm in diameter, preferably with C-shaped flexible

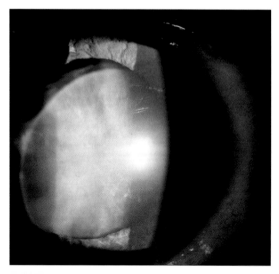

FIGURE 17–7. Large zonular dyalisis (between 7 and 1 o'clock).

loops, will be indicated and can be placed in-the-bag without major difficulty. A flexible acrylic lens may also be a good option.

According to Apple and collaborators, intraocular silicone lenses should not be implanted in situations where the possibility of retina detachment and a possible repair using silicone oil may be foreseen. In the absence of the posterior capsule, this silicone oil will tend to adhere to the surface of the intraocular lens, adversely affecting its optical qualities and consequently causing a considerable reduction in visual acuity.[4]

In presence of an extensive capsular rupture greater than 70%, our preference will be to use the remainder of the anterior lens capsule to hold a lens placed in the ciliary sulcus. In these cases, a 14 mm diameter lens with more rigid loops will provide additional safety at this location. Should there be any doubt regarding the stability of the implant, the lens may be iris-fixated with a 10–0 Prolene suture.

In cases of perforating injuries, the ruptured anterior and posterior lens capsules tend to induce fibrosis. This may cause a concentric traction at the base of the vitreous, with an eventual retinal detachment. Attention should be given to these patients during the first few postoperative years, monitoring the condition of the retina and if necessary, YAG-laser may be indicated to reduce or eliminate the traction forces caused by the fibrosis present.

In the presence of a cataract and retinal detachment, a lensectomy may be performed at a later date. Priority is given to correcting the retina, provided the lens opacification will allow a safe repair. In cases of vitreous hemorrhage or choroidal detachment, observation for few days may allow easier clot removal.

In cases where a repaired cornea presents intense edema, consider waiting a few days until its transparency is sufficient to allow a safe lensectomy. This approach will depend on whether or not there is uveitis or an increased intraocular pressure present.

Phacoemulsification or phacoaspiration can be very helpful in solving cases of traumatic cataracts. It allows better control over the surgical procedure through a small incision. Only adjustments in regard to the flow rate, vacuum and ultrasound power will be required, to prevent a possible expansion of a posterior capsular rupture, and displacement of the cataract into the vitreous body. In general, these three parameters should be reduced during the surgery.

■ Tips and Pearls

1. Evaluate the level of involvement and find the cause of the trauma.
2. Always consider the presence of an intraocular foreign body if a perforation is present. In perforating injuries, the posterior capsule might be compromised.
3. Block the facial nerve to prevent further loss of the intraocular contents if a major injury is present. If you suspect an extensive corneal/scleral laceration and there is severe lid edema making an appropriate exam difficult, handle this under general anesthesia.
4. Determine if the injury can be handled under local or general anesthesia.
5. If a total cataract is present, the main challenge will be the capsulorhexis. Handle it as an intumescent cataract.
6. A complete anterior lens luxation is treated by intracapsular lensectomy and an AC IOL implantation after vitrectomy. A scleral-fixated IOL is considered when an AC IOL is not indicated.
7. If less than 45 degrees of subluxation is present, phacoemulsification is performed as the usual manner. Basically will be a phacoaspiration after a good hydrodissection.
8. If the dialysis is more than 45 degrees and less than 180, choose your entrance carefully, consider using the endocapsular ring after a careful CCC. Use low flow, low vacuum, and power settings for the surgery. If there is more than 180 degrees of zonular dehiscence, an intracapsular lensectomy will be indicated.
9. If a ruptured posterior capsule is suspected as a result of the injury, a liberal use of viscoelastics and a dry aspiration will be indicated.

10. Remember to perform all repairs at a single setting if possible, e.g., repairing the corneal/scleral laceration, removal of the intraocular foreign body if present, cataract extraction, anterior and posterior vitrectomy if needed, and IOL implantation. This will contribute to a better recovery of this traumatized eye. Always consider a PMMA IOL implantation if further retina work will be needed.

REFERENCES

1. Rezende F, Pinheiro Dias JF. Trauma Ocular in Contro-vérsias & Complicações em cirurgia ocular. Editora Cultura Médica, Rio de Janeiro, 1996.
2. Fukuhara M, Kosaka T, Fujitake S. Intraocular foreign body discovered after cataract extraction. Folia Ophtalmol Jpn 1991;42:1399–1401.
3. Stegman, R. Manejo de la catarata traumática. In: Boyd B (ed). Highlights of Ophthalmology 1995;6(6):76–78.
4. Apple DJ, Federman JL, Krolicki TJ, et al. Irreversible silicone oil adhesion to silicone intraocular lenses. Ophthalmology 1996;103:1555–1562.

18

Phacoemulsification in Severe Chronic Obstructive Pulmonary Disease

I. HOWARD FINE AND RICHARD S. HOFFMAN

The transition from extracapsular cataract extraction to phacoemulsification has greatly reduced the intraoperative risks of performing cataract surgery in patients with chronic obstructive pulmonary disease (COPD). Faster operating times and small, 3 mm self-sealing incisions have made cataract surgery more comfortable and safer in these patients. Despite this, there are special considerations which should be made in COPD patients to assist in the best possible outcomes. This is especially true when cataract surgery may be prolonged because of concomitant glaucoma, corneal, or vitreous surgery. The two main obstacles to overcome when performing cataract surgery in COPD patients are coughing and intolerance to the fully supine position.

■ Cough

Most patients may undergo surgery under topical anesthesia; however, patients with severe COPD who may be prone to frequent coughing might benefit from local anesthesia in order to reduce the risk of choroidal hemorrhage or effusion. In most instances, coughing during phacoemulsification is not problematic since surgical instruments can be removed from the eye at the first hint of a cough. The small incision should self seal maintaining the integrity of the intraocular contents. In most instances of coughing, it may be preferable to leave the phacoemulsification probe in the eye in foot position 1 in order to maintain pressure within the globe. The forehead should be supported with the second hand reducing the risks from excessive head movement.

Preoperative medications can assist in cough elimination or suppression. Bronchodilators administered by nebulizer or aerosol treatments help patients with severe COPD clear bronchial secretions long enough to eliminate coughing during surgery. Albuterol 2.5 mg. (0.5 ml of the 0.5% solution diluted with 2.5 cc sterile normal saline) delivered over 10 minutes by nebulizer or two puffs of Albuterol inhalation aerosol administered 30 minutes prior to surgery have been extremely effective in alleviating coughing in even the most recalcitrant COPD patient. Cough suppressants in the form of dextromethorphan cough lozenges and cough syrup are also extremely helpful. If the need arises to suppress the cough reflex during the procedure, fentanyl 25–50 µg or lidocaine 20 mg can be administered intravenously.

■ Oxygen Therapy

Oxygen administration by nasal cannula is employed during surgery for all cataract patients. In patients with COPD, low flow oxygen administration at 1 to 3 liters per minute is the usual dose. Oxygen flows higher than this are feared to place the patient at risk for worsening hypercapnia; however, we do not feel this is a problem for the short duration of increased oxygen administration which may occur during phacoemulsification.

■ Positioning for Surgery

Most patients with COPD can undergo surgery lying flat on an operating table. Positioning the patient with pillows under the legs and shoulders with the bed in a slight Trendelenberg position is helpful in maintaining patient comfort by simulating the sitting position.

There are many patients with severe COPD who find it almost impossible to assume a supine position. It is possible to perform phacoemulsification in a patient who is not fully supine. Rimmer and Miller[1] previously reported on a case of phacoemulsification performed in the standing position. They used loupe magnification and headlamp illumination in order to remove a cataract in a patient unable to recline because of myotonic dystrophy and advanced interstitial lung disease. Other surgeons have also reported performing standing phacoemulsification using the operating microscope in patients who were unable to recline fully.[2,3]

Unfortunately, positioning a patient in a seated or partially reclined position creates an abnormal angle of approach for the operating room microscope which results in difficulty focusing and manipulating tissues and instruments intraocularly. Also, with the head in an upright position, gravity causes shallowing of the anterior chamber moving both the posterior capsule and the vitreous forward. This creates a greater risk for damaging the cornea and the posterior capsule during the procedure.

We have attempted to address the problems inherent in approaching these patients surgically by altering a waiting room chair to enable these patients to remain in an upright seated position and place their head back so that surgery can be performed in the usual head position obtained in the supine position on an operating room table (Figs. 18–1 to 18–3).

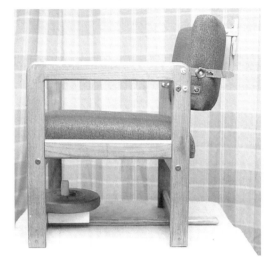

FIGURE 18–1. Waiting room chair altered by placing back cushion of chair on adjustable brackets. Legs shortened and head rest clamp attached to back of chair. Spindle for counterbalance weight attached to base. Chair in upright position.

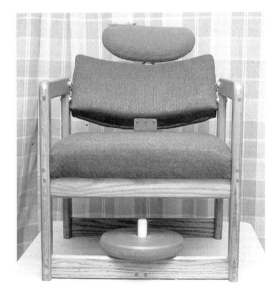

FIGURE 18–2. Front view of reclined chair with counterbalance weight between front legs.

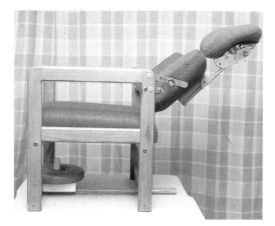

FIGURE 18–3. Side view of reclined chair.

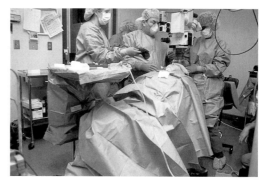

FIGURE 18–5. Claustrophobic patient undergoing cataract surgery with partial eye drape sitting in reclined chair.

We have operated on approximately 10 patients in this manner, all of them without complication or difficulty, and in some cases with somewhat greater ease for the surgeon because there was no limitation in head access. In each instance, patients were free of some of the congestive and anoxic symptoms they had in a supine position (Fig. 18–4).

There are occasional COPD patients who are also unable to tolerate a full face surgical drape because of claustrophobia. We have found it useful in these patients to perform a full face preparation and use only an aperture drape around the eye; avoiding draping the rest of the face so that the sensation of being closed in was eliminated (Fig. 18–5).

■ **Phacoemulsification**

Phacoemulsification in COPD patients is performed the same as in any other patient. The use of cracking or chopping techniques within an epinuclear shell allows for added safety should the patient move or cough. Special attention should be directed at removing all viscoelastic material at the conclusion of the procedure since the treatment of postoperative pressure increases is limited by the intolerance of COPD patients to many glaucoma medications. Nonselective beta blockers should be avoided and even selective beta blockers should be used cautiously since many severe COPD patients will cross react to beta 1 blockers, worsening their respiratory function.

■ **Conclusion**

Cataract surgery continues to undergo improvements and refinements making it safer and faster. Although most patients with chronic obstructive pulmonary disease can undergo phacoemulsification without regards to their respiratory disease, patients with severe pulmonary disease often present challenges to the cataract surgeon. Coughing will usually present itself as more of a nuisance than a threat to surgical outcome now that incision architecture has allowed for small self-sealing wounds. Despite this, there are measures that can be taken preoperatively to help

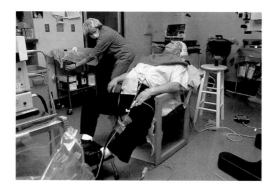

FIGURE 18–4. Patient with chronic obstructive pulmonary disease reclining comfortably in chair prior to undergoing cataract surgery. Legs resting on foot rest.

reduce the incidence of coughing allowing for safer uninterrupted phacoemulsification.

Probably the greatest obstacle and challenge for performing surgery in these patients are those individuals who are unable to fully recline for the operation. Phacoemulsification can be performed in the standing position to accommodate patients who are intolerant to the supine position, however, we feel that new surgical tables and/or surgical chairs will allow patients with severe COPD to undergo phacoemulsification under safer and more comfortable conditions in the future.

■ Tips and Pearls

1. Patients prone to coughing during cataract surgery should have small self-sealing incisions for maintaining the integrity of the intraocular contents.
2. In most instances of coughing, it may be preferable to leave the phacoemulsification probe in the eye in foot position 1 in order to maintain pressure within the globe.
3. Bronchodilators administered by nebulizer or aerosol treatments help patients with severe COPD clear bronchial secretions long enough to eliminate coughing during surgery.
4. If the need arises to suppress the cough reflex during the procedure, fentanyl 25–50 μg or lidocaine 20 mg can be administered intravenously.
5. An altered waiting room chair which allows patients to remain in an upright seated position and place their head back can enable surgery to be performed more comfortably in patients with severe chronic obstructive pulmonary disease.

REFERENCES

1. Rimmer S, Miller KM. Phacoemulsification in the standing position with loupe magnification and headlamp illumination. J Cataract Refract Surg 1994;20: 353–354.
2. Hunter LH. Standing while performing phacoemulsification. J Cataract Refract Surg 1995;21:111.
3. Liu C. Phacoemulsification in a patient with torticollis. J Cataract Refract Surg 1995;21:364.

19

Phacoemulsification in Patients with Bleeding Disorders

HORACIO U. ROTMAN, JOHN BELARDO, ANA C. SANSEAU, AND LUIS W. LU

Cataract surgery is mainly performed among the elderly, in which a number of systemic conditions are more frequent. Cataract surgery, anesthesia, and postoperative care involve a very low risk due to the advancements of surgical techniques. However, many factors including cardiovascular, renal, hepatic, rheumatologic, and bleeding disorders may alter the normal process of hemostasis.

The above abnormalities and the drugs used to treat them may also have effects on hemostasis and coagulation.

Blood dyscrasia is an old term used in reference to both plasma and blood cell abnormalities. Currently, they are widely known as bleeding disorders (Table 19–1). The ophthalmologist should be fully aware of the effects bleeding disorders may produce during cataract surgery.[1,2]

The use of clear corneal incisions has changed the way we look at patients on anti-coagulation therapy. In a patient in whom the cornea is clear, the pupil dilates well, and the anterior chamber is of normal depth, the risks are minimal. Average phaco skills should not pose any untoward challenges. For a beginning surgeon, anti-coagulation therapy is a potential danger and should be discontinued in preparation for surgery.

Cataract surgery performed at the limbus with minimal or no conjunctival manipulation can be performed without interruption of anticoagulation therapy. The same holds true for clear corneal incisions which avoid blood vessels at the limbus or conjunctiva. Longer scleral tunnels, however, do run a risk of bleeding both intra and postoperatively.

Anticoagulants should be discontinued in complicated cataract surgery where there is a need to manipulate the iris or place a scleral fixation suture. Anterior chamber disruption with shallow anterior chambers, ruptured or irregular iris with anterior synechea, and traumatic cataracts with loose zonules require special considerations and flexibility intraoperatively which cannot be planned for every time. A patient who has continued anticoagulants and develops intra-operative complete zonular dehiscence will not be a candidate for scleral fixation sutures. If this same patient were not a candidate for an anterior chamber-intraocular lens (AC-IOL) the patient may have to undergo yet another procedure off the anticoagulants exposing him/her to a potential choroidal hemorrhage, endophthalmitis, epithelial downgrowth, and all the other unmentionables associated with complicated intraocular procedures. Preoperative evaluation and surgical planning is fundamental to success and avoidance of poor outcomes.

It should be emphasized there is no need to know every hematologic pathology in depth. The physician should identify the group the patient belongs to in order to decide which

Table 19–1. Bleeding Disorders: Hemorrhagic Diatheses

Increased vascular fragility.
Reduced platelet number
    Thrombocytopenia
Defective platelet function.
Abnormalities in the clotting factors
    Deficiencies of factor VII - v WF complex
    Factor IX deficiency (Christmas disease, hemophilia B)
Disseminated intravascular coagulation (DIC)
Derived from systemic diseases
    Hepatic disease
    Presence of lupic anticoagulant
    Uremic disease

laboratory tests should be required and to foresee the management of any complication that may arise. Therefore, the disorders have been split into three major groups according to the cellular type involved.

1. Red Cell Diseases. They seldom produce considerable bleeding except for those associated with neoplasms (i.e. Pernicious Anemia, Polycythemia Vera).

2. White Blood Cell Diseases. Benign primary alterations of these cells do not imply modifications in the course of action. White cell lines may be involved in malignant processes and hemostasis is modified. Examples of this are the Myelodysplastic Syndromes, as they modify the megakaryocite line preventing platelet formation. Other examples include Acute Leukemia and Chronic Myelogenous Leukemia.

3. Hemostasis Disorders. They include all those pathologies that are due to the alteration of platelets, vessels, or coagulation factors involved in the coagulation pathways (Fig. 19–1 and 19–2), causing bleeding. The clinical signs include purpura, ecchymosis, and petechiae. Examples of hemostasis disorders include Hemophilia, Multiple Myeloma, Schonlein-Henoch Purpura, Idiopathic Thrombocytopenic Purpura, and poor coagulation due to lack of vitamin K.

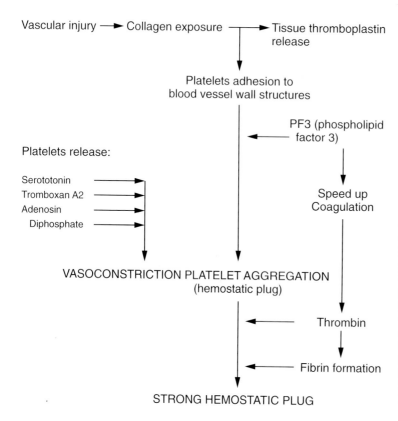

FIGURE 19–1. Hemostasis and platelet interaction with coagulation. After a vascular injury with endothelial destruction, the collagen fibers are exposed. In response, platelets become adhesive. Isolated platelets come in contact and are exposed to PF3, attaining the primary platelet plug. Platelets release ADP, serotonin, and TX A2, inducing vasoconstriction while PF3 speeds up the coagulation process and the generation of thrombin and fibrin which will contribute to the stabilization of the platelet plug.[3]

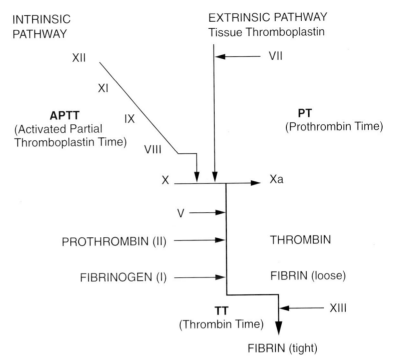

FIGURE 19–2. Coagulation process. The extrinsic pathway starts with tissue thromboplastin, which interacts with factor VII to convert factor X to factor Xa and start the common final pathway. The intrinsic pathway needs the interaction of factors, XII, XI, IX, and VIII to convert factor X to Xa. The common final pathway involves factor, X, V, II (prothrombin), and I (fibrinogen). The coagulation final product is fibrin. Factor XIII (fibrin stabilizing factor) converts fibrin to a more stable state.[3]

■ Preliminary Patient Evaluation and Preparation

Medical History

A detailed medical history describing a personal background should be obtained in order to take into account frequent bleedings (Fig.

Table 19–2. Drug-Induced Hemostasis Alteration (most representative drugs)

By Interfering with platelet function
Salicilates: nonsalicylates; antibiotics (penicillins, cephalosporins, chloramphericol); Ticlopidine; Dypiridamole
Anticoagulants
  Heparin
Mode of action: By acting jointly with antithrombin-III it inhibits factors in the coagulation process (intrinsic and common pathways).
  Vitamin K antagonists: hydroxycoumarin, warfarin, acenocoumarol, dicoumarol.
Mode of action: They prevent the production of vitamin K dependent factors altering the extrinsic pathway.
Miscellaneous
  Anticonvulsants: diphenylhydantoin, carbamazepine, valproic acid
  Diuretics : chlorothiazide, furosemide
  Quinidine, Alpha-methyldopa, ranitidine, sulfonamides, rifampin
Mode of action: Inmunologic mechanism thrombocytopenia.

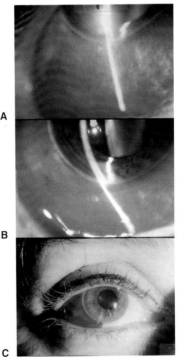

FIGURE 19–3. Subconjuctival hemorrhage. **(A,B)** Patient with abnormal clotting factors. **(C)** Young woman with vasculopathy.

19–3), important and long-lasting hematomas produced by minor trauma, bleeding time, medication type dosage, and frequency of medicines administered and all systemic diseases that may affect hemostasis (Table 19–2).

It is often necessary to mention the medication to the patient, especially aspirin, NSAIDS, minor sedatives (benzodiazepines), antihistamines, and anti-inflammatory preparations which are over the counter and not usually perceived as real drugs to patients. It is also important to explore the family history for bleeding disorders which could alert the ophthalmologist to use extra precautions both preoperatively and intraoperatively.

Physical Examination

Physical examination may be misleading as no signs may be present during the exam; however, bleeding disorders can be found through routine preoperative screening blood work (Table 19–3). Petechiae are typical in platelet disorders, while ecchymosis characterizes the alterations in the coagulation pathways.

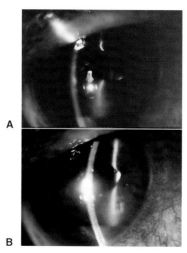

FIGURE 19–4 (A, B). Postoperative hyphema in a patient with bleeding disorder.

Table 19–3. Laboratory Tests

PROTHROMBIN TIME (PT)
Tests extrinsic and common pathways
Normal value: 12 seconds
Abnormal values detect vitamin K dependent factors deficiency, hepatic disease, DIC, oral anticoagulants
ACTIVATED PARTIAL THROMBOPLASTIN TIME (APTT)
Tests intrinsic and common pathways.
Normal value: 25 to 40 seconds
Abnormal values suggest disorders such as hemophilia, Von Willebrand disease, heparin therapy, DIC, factors SII, IS and S deficiency, circulating anticoagulants.
THROMBIN TIME (TT)
Tests the conversion of fibrinogen to fibrin.
Normal value: 10 to 15 seconds
Abnormal values indicate third phase coagulation pathology, DIC, fibrin aggregation products, severe hypofibrinogenemia.
BLEEDING TIME (BT)
Tests primary hemostasis, that is platelet function.
Normal values: 3 to 7 minutes
Abnormal values indicate platelet disorder, Von Willebrand disease, thrombocytopenia.

Note: Should these tests results be normal, no serious hemorrhagic diathesis is likely to be present. Any abnormality indicates that research should be carried out to detect specific defects. Such evaluation should be made by a specialized team experienced with hematologic pathology in order to undertake the studies in a reasonable way.

Preparing the Patient for Surgery

All those potentially antiaggregative or anticoagulant drugs may be discontinued a week prior to surgery under medical supervision provided that no contraindications are reported. Topical antiprostaglandin is not given prior to surgery since there exists the potential for increased bleeding time due to interference with thrombocyte aggregation.

The Phacoemulsification techniques that the surgeon commands should be varied. You may have your favorite technique which befalls the majority of cataracts mercilessly. However, every situation and cataract demands a variation of that same technique and a completely different approach at times. In the anticoagulated patient you would want to avoid any manipulations that bring your phaco tip close to the iris thus increasing the risk for iris trauma (Fig. 19–4). Anterior chamber, iris plane, and in-the-bag phaco can all be performed safely in the hands of a careful surgeon who takes extra care to avoid iris injury or excessive conjunctival manipulation.[5] The small pupil need not be an absolute contra-indication. It presents a challenge in the hands of experienced phaco surgeons and it should not be performed by beginners if the patient is anticoagulated.

Most patients on anticoagulation medications have ischemia or diabetes with accompanying floppy and atrophic irides. This makes their cases particularly challenging. Patients with Fuchs' dystrophy have fine vessels on their iris surface that may bleed during the procedure (Amsler' sign). The bleeding seen with this condition is usually minimal but can pose a problem with anticoagulants.

■ Surgical Considerations

Anesthesia

Topical anesthesia and intravenous sedation are preferred, if not contraindicated. General anesthesia, is necessary in cases when topical or local anesthesia is not indicated. No ocular block is necessary. Local anesthesia, such as retrobulbar and peribulbar anesthesia, is relatively contraindicated in patients with bleeding disorders. When topical anesthesia is indicated, careful patient selection is essential.[6] Proparacaine (0.5% one drop every 2 minutes x 2 at the pre-op holding area); Marcaine (0.75% without epinephrine every 3 minutes x 4) is given. Tetracaine (0.5%) may be used or topical Xylocaine without epinephrine. The schedule is repeated again prior to transfer to the operating room, once the patient is on the operating table, and when is being prepped for surgery.

It has been noted that marcaine is the least toxic to the epithelium. You may want to make note of your patients with a history of eye trauma, corneal abrasion, anterior basement membrane dystrophy, or recurrent corneal erosion to minimize the number of anesthetic drops given and choosing topical marcaine instead.

Topical anesthesia can be performed with or without intravenous sedation. Intravenous sedation can make it difficult for patients to control their eye movement. Sublingual versed can be administered if necessary. Sublingual versed does not have the respiratory depression that is found with IV administration. Careful patient selection is essential. Intracameral administration of nonpreserved 1% lidocaine is an excellent adjunct in topical anesthesia. Some surgeons prefer to deliver this in a 50–50 dilution with BSS during the hydrodissection of the lens. This is felt to be less challenging to the endothelium as the solution is buffered and the patient does not experience any discomfort as with full strength lidocaine. If hydrodissection is not performed, viscoelastic in the A/C protects the endothelium before injecting the full strength lidocaine into the A/C.

In patients with bleeding disorders, some of the benefits of a clear corneal incision are as follows:

1. The conjunctiva is not touched, therefore, no subjunctival bleeding is observed.
2. Cauterization is not needed. Cauterization of conjunctival vessels increases the probability of early postoperative bleeding and wound leakage.
3. Faster visual recovery. Patients are able to monitor their vision in the immediate postop period when IOP spikes can occur and call their physician.
4. Faster and less traumatic than a scleral pocket incision. No postoperative hyphemas.
5. Astigmatism correction may be managed by selecting the incision site or a temporally placed incision that would be astigmatically neutral.

Incision

Taking into consideration that patients with most hematologic disorders tend to bleed easily, *our indication for these patients shall be clear corneal incision.* A 2.6 mm incision is performed for the Mackool tip; a 2.5 mm incision for the Storz microseal needle (which can be used on most phaco machines); a 2.8 mm for the microtip; or a 3.00 mm for the regular tip of the Legacy phacoemulsification unit. Dr. Charles Williamson is now using a 1.9 mm incision with the microflow needle and inserting a new Staar lens through the same incision (personal communication). The incision is performed without conjunctival manipulation. The Fine-Thornton ring for fixation, is avoided. No bridle sutures are applied.

Fixation of the globe should not be performed with instruments that manipulate the conjunctiva (Fig. 19–5). Fixation can be achieved with an iris spatula or with the cystotome needle. The valve incision is performed either with a diamond or metal 2.5 mm keratome in a two-step fashion (Fig. 19–6). First the incision is made through the epithelium and into the stroma traveling approximately 1.5 to 2.0

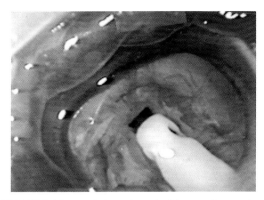

FIGURE 19–5. Subconjunctival hemorrhage during cataract surgery in a patient with anticoagulation therapy with heparin.

mm. The blade is then directed downwards piercing Descemet's membrane and entering the anterior chamber. If you maintain at least a 2 mm stromal tunnel you will avoid iris prolapse and wound leakage. The capsulotomy can be performed with the cystotome needle through the paracentesis wound or with capsulotomy forceps through the 2.5 mm incision. As soon as you enter the anterior chamber, viscoeslastic is injected deepening and protecting the iris and anterior capsule from any injury which can easily occur if the patient were to move the eye in the wrong direction.

With the patient looking at the light, a large continuous curvilinear capsulotomy is performed. The procedure is performed under low to moderate illumination. This makes it easier for the patient to adapt to the light and cooperate with instructions. Low to moderate light intensity should be sufficient to safely perform the procedure without compromising visualization.

Phacoemulsification Technique

The phaco snap procedure using the phaco chopper while impaling the nucleus with the phaco tip for fixation is an excellent procedure for most cataracts. The snapping procedure makes use of the pulsed phaco power which transmits a shock wave through the core of the cataract. The chopper instrument nudges slightly in a tangential direction towards the phaco tip cracking the nucleus without having to drag the chopper through the length of the lens. Depending on the hardness of the cataract the chopping or snapping would be minimal, two pieces for softer cataracts or 6 to 8 for dense cataracts. The smaller sized pupils lend themselves to chopping into small pieces. Once they are removed from the bag and brought into the central anterior chamber, safe phacoemulsification can be performed (Fig. 19–7).

It is critical that the phaco system you use does not produce an anterior chamber trampoline. A stable chamber is a reliable and safe area to work in. Any technique you use must have a safe area in which you can maneuver in the event the patient moves the eye. With the phaco tip and chopper in the eye, most eye movements are under the surgeon's control. The epinucleus can be easily tumbled and aspirated with the phaco tip and if necessary, very low power or short pulses of phaco are used. The iris spatula can be used to manipulate the epinucleus. The larger the capsulotomy the easier it is to remove.

Removing cortex is as varied as the terrain. A large capsulotomy obviously makes removal

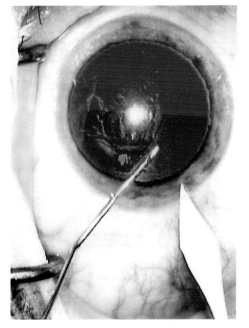

FIGURE 19–6. Clear cornea valve incision with fixation of globe with cystotome needle attached to viscoelastic after completion of capsulotomy through paracentesis wound.

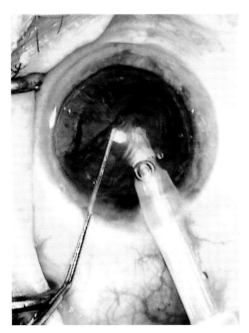

FIGURE 19–7. Phaco snap through a 2.5 mm incision using the Storz Microflow needle and the Allergan Diplomax phacoemulsification unit.

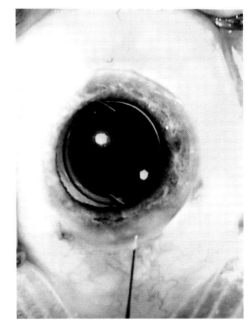

FIGURE 19–8. Allergan SI-40 IOL in position. Hydration of wound at end of procedure with BSS and Lidocaine 1 % in 50/50 mix.

much easier. Smaller capsulotomies tend to hug the cortex and not let it go. Straight cannulas with silicone sleeves through a 2.5 mm incision give you a deep and safe chamber where even subincisional cortex can be removed safely. All metal I A cannulas through a 2.5 mm incision also maintain chamber very well. The 45 degree angled tip allows for easy access to subincisional as well as other quadrants. Sticky cortex can be loosened using the reflex mode with the I A cannula. Dual port I A is also an excellent and safer alternative to remove cortex. Stubborn nonmoving cortex can be left alone and after IOL insertion can be safely removed using the IOL to protect the bag (Fig. 19–8). The IOL can also be rotated on the bag which allows the haptics to physically sweep and loosen the stubborn cortex. Remember, a little bit of cortex is better than a little vitrectomy! IOL insertion before cortex removal should be considered in the following patients (1) status postvitrectomy; (2) high myopia (or any situation where the capsule is flopping around exhibiting no tension or stability; and (3) small posterior capsular rent without vitreous prolapse (placing the lens protects the capsule from tearing further while placing a physical barrier between the anterior chamber fluids and vitreous).

In-the-bag phacoemulsification techniques are preferred preventing damage to the iris which would produce immediate bleeding during and after surgery. It is advisable to refrain from administering subjunctval antibiotic and corticosteroid injections to prevent a subconjunctival hemorrhage. In some patients with prosthetic heart valves, recent cardiovascular surgery or preventive therapy for deep venous thrombosis, anticoagulant suspension is contraindicated.

■ Postoperative Considerations

All analgesics that may modify hemostasis are contraindicated. We recommend the administration of Acetaminophen or Lysine Chlorohydrate since these drugs do not alter the coagulation values. Propoxiphen is contraindicated in patients with bleeding disorders due to the possibility of an immunologic thrombocytopenia. In the overwhelming majority of patients undergoing topical anesthesia, seldom if ever does a patient require pain medication. Most patients experience a slight foreign body sensation which they tolerate well. However, in the event you need to manage a corneal abrasion our experience with PRK serves us well.

A bandage contact lens—either silicone or collagen—would be appropriate management. The benefits of a bandage contact lens (BCL) include: covering the epithelial defect so that the blinking of the lids does not interfere with epithelial repair therefore avoids patching the eye. BCL increases the delivery of antibiotics and anti-inflammatory eye drops to the anterior chamber. The most superior delivery system to the anterior chamber (A/C) other than direct injection into the A/C is topical drops. BCL augments this delivery system. The use of nonsteroidal anti-inflammatory drops also helps greatly with analgesia. This innovation has changed the face of PRK postoperative pain management. In the case of a slow, clear corneal wound leak with a well formed chamber, a BCL aids in tamponading and healing of the wound. We would also recommend an eye shield until the leak is sealed. In the event there is a need for a BCL, the patient can still monitor their vision and alert the physician for sudden loss of vision which may be due to increased IOP. The problem can be addressed earlier rather then the next day if they were patched thus avoiding the potential or a vessel occlusion or ischemia.[7]

■ Tips and Pearls

The risk of surgical bleeding in predisposed patients may be diminished if these guidelines are followed:

1. Determine the type of coagulopathy. Stop administration of drugs that can modify hemostasis in the pre- and postoperative period. Do not use NSAIDS nor propoxiphen.
2. We prefer topical anesthesia and a clear corneal incision. In-the-bag phacoemulsification is the preferred technique. Remember not to use subconjunctival injections.
3. Request a hematological consult whenever required.
4. Surgical outcomes are best planned for by a careful and thorough preoperative evaluation. The decision to perform topical anesthesia should be a conscious endeavor that includes not only the ocular structures but the physical and mental status of our patients.

REFERENCES

1. Hay A, Olsen K, Nicholson DH. Bleeding complications in thrombocytopenic patients undergoing ophthalmic surgery. Am J Ophthalmol 1990;109:482–483.
2. Cunningham RD. Retinopathy of blood dyscrasias. In: Tasman W, Yaeger EA (eds). Duane's Clinical Ophthalmology. Philadelphia: JB Lippincott; 1994;:1–8.
3. Rozman C, Montserrat E. Hematologia. In: Farreras P, Rozman C (eds). Medicina Interna. Barcelona: Marin; 1992;271–301.
4. Fraunfelder FT. Drug-Induced Ocular Side Effects. Baltimore: Williams & Wilkins; 1996;12–52.
5. Jaffe NS. Cataract Surgery and its Complications. St. Louis: CV Mosby; 1976;321–340.
6. Fine IH, Fichman RA, Grabow HB. Clear-Corneal Cataract Surgery and Topical Anesthesia. Thorofare NJ: Slack; 1993; 97–167.
7. McMeel JW. Uveal Tract Circulatory Problems. In: Albert DM, Jacobiec FA (eds). Principles and Practice of Ophthalmology. Philadelphia: WB Saunders; 1994; 389–396.

20

Phacoemulsification in the Presence of Neovascularization of the Iris

EHUD I. ASSIA

Neovascularization of the iris (Rubeosis Iridis), is an evidence and a result of retinal ischemia, usually caused by diabetes mellitus or vascular occlusive disease. The treatment of neovascularization is by intense and controlled destruction of the ischemic retina by laser panretinal photocoagulation (PRP) or by cryoablation (PRC). In both cases, direct visualization of the retina is required to assure sufficient and effective treatment. However, in some cases a dense cataract may develop and obscure the retinal visualization. Cataract removal is then indicated, not only to improve the patient's visual function, but also to allow an immediate and effective retinal ablation.[1] Prompt treatment is often necessary to prevent further development of neovascularization and subsequent severe complications such as traction retinal detachment and neovascular glaucoma.[2-4] Cataract extraction is thus performed in the presence of severe and active iris neovascularization.[5] Insult to the fragile blood vessels may cause intraoperative bleeding which significantly complicates surgery, and may cause intraocular pressure rise or further delay retinal photocoagulation. Neovascularization is often accompanied by posterior synechia and a peripupillary membrane. However, synechiolysis and membrane removal may also result in extensive bleeding.

A technique to remove the cataract by phacoemulsification and minimize intraoperative bleeding is herein described.

■ Preoperative Evaluation

Evaluation of the lens opacity and the density of the cataract is often difficult because of a constricted pupil, the presence of posterior synechiae and/or corneal edema. Hard nucleus may require a prolonged surgical time and a high ultrasonic energy, however, phacoemulsification is advantageous since the lens material can be removed through a relatively small pupil, whereas forceful stretching of the pupil during manual extraction may increase the risk of intraoperative bleeding.

Preoperative evaluation of the posterior segment is also very important. The rate of neovascular formation in the anterior segment, as well as of the retinal neovascularization, determines the surgical urgency and priority. Neovascularization that progresses despite prior extensive retinal photocoagulation is associated with very poor prognosis. If the retina is not adequately observed, B scan ultrasonography is effective in detecting the presence of a retinal detachment or vitreous hemorrhage. Evaluation of visual function by electroretinogram (ERG) and visually evoked potential (VEP) is sometimes of value to predict the final visual potential.

Ocular neovascularization almost always requires early retinal treatment in addition to lens removal, such as repair of a retinal detachment and/or intraoperative endolaser photocoagulation.[6,7] A team of anterior and posterior segment surgeons in the same surgical setting is often required.

■ Surgical Technique

The primary concern of the surgeon is to prevent and if possible, eliminate intraoperative bleeding (Fig. 20–1). This can be accomplished by direct coagulation of the iridal blood vessels by using intraocular cautery (Fig. 20–2). Since heat is generated during diathermy, a cooling system is then required. This is effectively achieved by continuous fluid irrigation using an anterior chamber maintainer (ACM). I have also found the ACM very useful also in routine cataract surgery because it maintains the anterior chamber volume and pressure throughout the operation, as well as in the surgical stages when the phaco probe is out of the eye. In complicated surgeries, and especially in the presence of iris neovascularization, the ACM is extremely valuable. The ACM is placed in the infero-temporal limbal area; inferiorly to keep it away from the surgical instruments, and temporal to keep it away from the nose.

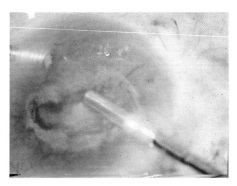

FIGURE 20–2. Cauterization of the pupillary margin using intraocular diathermy. The energy is set to create bleaching of the iris. Some of the large vessels may require individual localized treatment. Continuous irrigation through the anterior chamber maintainer allows safe intraocular manipulations and serves as a cooling system.

Coagulation of the iris blood vessels is performed by using intraocular diathermy inserted through a 1.2 to 1.5 mm paracentesis incision. The cautery should be adjusted to form blanching of the treated area, yet to avoid excessive damage to the iris which may result in tissue necrosis. The initial treatment is applied to the pupillary margin for 360 degrees, followed by coagulation of the large blood vessels. Usually it is not necessary to cauterize the entire iris surface, even if the neovascularization is extensive. In most cases, limited diathermy at the pupillary margin is

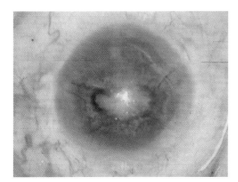

FIGURE 20–1. Extensive neovascularization of the iris in a diabetic patient. The constricted pupil is covered by a richly vascularized fibrous membrane, except over a small area of ectropion uvea.

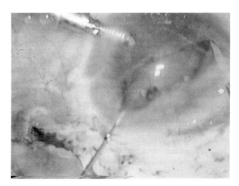

FIGURE 20–3. Stretching of the pupil with two instruments in an X motion after coagulation of the pupillary margin all around. Note that no bleeding occurs.

CHAPTER 20 ■ Neovascularization of the Iris

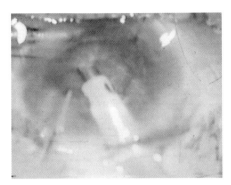

FIGURE 20–4. The inferior half of the pupil is enlarged with two flexible iris dilators. Phacoemulsification is performed by the "stop & chop" technique. Using cracking techniques, phacoemulsification is done at the center, avoiding contact with the iris.

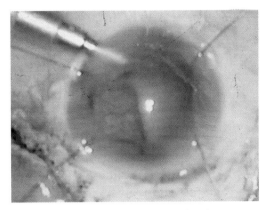

FIGURE 20–6. After lens removal a dense retrolenticular vascularized membrane is seen on the left and a yellow reflex of a tractional retinal detachment is seen on the right, behind the posterior capsule. Surgery was continued by the vitreo-retinal surgeon.

sufficient to forcefully stretch and enlarge the constricted pupil and even to cut and remove vascularized membranes (Fig. 20–3). If the pupil is not adequately enlarged, pupil dilators are sometimes necessary, however, they should be placed gently and carefully to avoid excessive tension over the pupillary border (Fig. 20–4).

Phacoemulsification is performed in the regular fashion. Cracking techniques are preferred since the separated pieces are brought to the center of the surgical field, avoiding the phaco probe to be in contact with the iris and the fragile blood vessels. Irrigation and aspiration should also be done cautiously because the I/A probe is inserted behind the iris to remove the cortical material from the capsular bag periphery. Since continuous irrigation is provided by the ACM, controlled and gentle aspiration can be done by using a thin 0.4 mm port cannula attached to a 5 cc syringe (Fig. 20–5).

Foldable lenses can be implanted easily through a small corneal incision, however, these complicated eyes often require retinal surgery including silicone oil injection (Fig. 20–6). Recent studies have shown that silicone oil and silicone lenses are not a good match, therefore solid PMMA lenses may be more appropriate. Since it may be necessary to perform PRP soon after the surgery, it might be better to suture the external incisions, even if under normal conditions the same incisions could have been left unsutured.

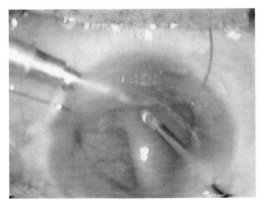

FIGURE 20–5. Aspiration of the cortical material with a 0.4 mm pore cannula is gentle and cautious. The irrigation is provided by the ACM.

■ Postoperative Therapy

Diabetic and ischemic eyes may respond with a severe inflammatory reaction following surgical intervention. The abnormal vessels lack the physiological blood ocular barrier and therefore fibrin formation and abundant presence of flare and cells are often observed.[8,9] Intensive steroid therapy is therefore required. Topical steroid eye drops are given every hour for the first 1 to 2 postoperative days. It is also advisable to inject subconjunctival steroids at the end of the procedure. Ischemic eyes are also prone to ocular infection and postoperative antibiotics are indicated for at least 1 week.

Diabetic retinopathy may worsen after cataract surgery, especially in eyes with proliferative retinopathy. Macular edema may persist for over a year in 50% of the patients, and retinal neovascularization may develop quickly after surgery. A close follow up and early preventive or therapeutic intervention are necessary in these particular patients.

■ Tips and Pearls

1. Continuous irrigation through an anterior chamber maintainer facilitates surgery and also acts as a cooling system.
2. Coagulation of the pupillary margin and large vessels with the use of intraocular diathermy is usually sufficient to allow pupil manipulation and safe phacoemulsification.
3. If bleeding occurs, elevation of the BSS bottle will increase the intraocular pressure and may stop the bleeding. Otherwise, bleeders are located and cauterized.
4. Phacoemulsification using cracking techniques at the central part of the surgical field is preferred, avoiding any contact with the vascularized iris.

REFERENCES

1. Hykin PG, Gregson RM, Hamilton AM. Extracapsular cataract extraction in diabetes with rubeosis iridis. Eye 1992;6(3):296–299.
2. Diabetes Control and Complications Trial Research Group. Effect of intensive treatment on the development and progression of long-term complications in adolescents with insulin-dependent diabetes mellitus: diabetes control and complications trial. J Ped 1994; 125:177–188.
3. Diabetes Control and Complications Trial Research Group. The effect of intensive treatment of diabetes on the development and progression of long-term complications in insulin-dependent diabetes mellitus. N Eng J Med 1993;329:977–986.
4. Jampol LM, Ebroon DA, Goldbaum MH. Peripheral proliferative retinopathies: an update on angiogenesis, etiologies and management. Surv Ophthalmol 1994; 38:519–540.
5. Benson WE, Brown GC, Tasman W, et al. Extracapsular cataract extraction with placement of a posterior chamber lens in patients with diabetic retinopathy. Ophthalmology 1993;100(5):730–738.
6. Ullern M, Nicol JL, Ruellan YM, et al. Phacoemulsification by the anterior approach combined with vitreoretinal surgery. J Fr Ophthalmol 1993;16(5):320–324.
7. Mamalis N, Teske MP, Kreisler KR, et al. Phacoemulsification combined with pars plana vitrectomy. Ophthalmic Surg 1991;22(4):194–198.
8. Aiello LP, Avery RI, Arrigg PG, et al. Vascular endothelial growth factor in ocular fluid of patients with diabetic retinopathy and ocular retinal disorders. N Eng J Med 1994;331:1480–1487.
9. Pierce EA, Avery RI, Foley ED, et al. Vascular endothelial growth factor/vascular permeability factor expression in a mouse model of retinal neovascularization. Proc Natl Acad Sci USA 1995;92:905–909.

21

Phacoemulsification in Patients with High Risk of Choroidal Hemorrhage

GUILLERMO A. PEREIRA AND LUIS W. LU

The intraoperative suprachoroidal hemorrhage and the consequential expulsive hemorrhage that can occur, constitute the most serious complication in ocular surgery. The conversion to in-the-bag phacoemulsification has basically eliminated the occurrence of this condition.

■ Incidence

Fortunately, the incidence of this severe complication which in the majority of cases causes total loss of the visual function in the affected eye, is relatively low and varies according to different authors, between 0.05 and 0.4 %.[1,2] It has been generally said, with respect to this serious complication, that every ocular surgeon will face it at least once in his/her professional life time.

The incidence of limited acute intraoperative suprachoroidal hemorrhage (AISH) has been reported to be 1.2% in planned extracapsular cataract extraction (ECCE) by nucleus expression and 0.81% in phacoemulsification procedures using an iris plane superior nuclear pole prolapse technique.[3]

The introduction of capsulorhexis has basically eliminated the occurrence of this entity.

■ Causes

Expulsive hemorrhage is due to two principal causes, the choroidal hemorrhage and the massive choroidal effusion. In both cases, there is a rapid collection of blood/fluid in the suprachoroidal space, increasing the intraocular pressure. If the problem cannot be controlled quickly, it will provoke total expulsion of the intraocular contents through the operative incision.

Improved wound architecture has yielded to provide consistent self-sealing closure. This improved wound design and newer phacoemulsification techniques have contributed to the decreased incidence of suprachoroidal hemorrhage. Total expulsion of the intraocular contents has not been reported in the presence of a small incision self-sealing well constructed operative wound.

■ Pathogenesis

The choroidal hemorrhage generally begins from the short posterior ciliary arteries after they penetrate the globe through the sclera surrounding the optic nerve. Histopathologic studies reveal that in many cases, the cause of the hemorrhage is the rupture of necrotic areas in the wall of the vessels.[4] With respect to this, it is useful to remember some physiopathologic details related to choroidal vessels. First, these arteries and arterioles share histologic characteristics with those of the spleen with the frequent presence of hyaline enlargement and sclerosis of the middle vascular wall layer in the absence of general vascular illness.[5] Unlike other blood vessels that support a low external pressure, the intraocular vessels (both choroidal and retinal) are subjected to intraocular pressure, which can be around 20 mmHg, or even higher in cases of glaucoma and can even cause vascular collapse, especially at the level of the arterioles where the intravascular pressure drops considerably. The direct result of this phenomena will be a sluggish circulation at this level reducing the blood supply to the vascular walls. We may add the anatomical detail that the choroidal arterioles do not have vasa vasorum, and rely exclusively on diffusion for their nutrition.[6]

If we accept the mechanism of wall alteration to explain the occurrence of the suprachoroidal hemorrhage, all those patients who may show signs of altered vascular flow have to be considered as potentially susceptible to this complication. In this list, we must include arterial hypertension, glaucoma, generalized arteriosclerosis, high myopia, vascular fragility, and diabetes (Fig. 21-1). The risk factors identified and reported in a 1986 study of ECCE cases included advanced age, the presence of glaucoma with an axial length greater than 25.0 mm, and nucleus expression ECCE. A case-control study of risk factors for intraoperative suprachoroidal expulsive hemorrhage identified age, glaucoma, increased intraocular pressure, increased axial length and elevated intraoperative pulse as risk factors.[7] If a patient showed this complication in the first operated eye, it is necessary to consider the second eye to be at high risk.

The other cause of expulsive hemorrhage is the massive choroidal effusion described for the first time by Girard.[8] In this clinical entity, for reasons that are not clear, there exists a rapid collection of clear liquid in the supra-

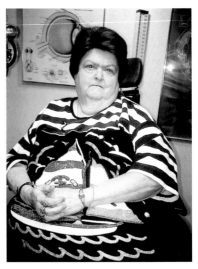

FIGURE 21–1. Seventy-five-year-old myopic patient with borderline controlled glaucoma, insulin-dependent diabetes, uncontrolled arterial hypertension, obesity, chronic obstructive pulmonary disease, and cataracts.

choroidal space, which can cause the same serious expulsive consequences as a choroidal hemorrhage.

There must be some additional unknown factors apart from the vascular alterations which have already been mentioned that can explain the occurrence of an expulsive hemorrhage. It has been accepted that outside factors exist such as inadequate local or general anesthesia and a sudden decrease of the intraocular pressure during cataract surgery, especially when predisposing factors are present.

In regard to phacoemulsification, the risk of suprachoroidal hemorrhage was present in former iris-plane phacoemulsification techniques in which the surgeon repeatedly prolapsed the superior pole of the nucleus into the anterior chamber for access by the phacoemulsification tip. This was accomplished by temporarily stopping the infusion so the relatively increased pressure in the vitreous cavity forced the superior pole forward. In capsular bag phacoemulsification, this maneuver is not necessary and the globe is always under pressure from the constant infusion flow and is spared the repeated pressure swings of the former iris plane techniques. It is believed that the improved fluid dynamic stability is primarily responsible for the decreased incidence of suprachoroidal hemorrhage at the present time.[3]

■ Clinical Manifestations

Expulsive hemorrhage usually happens during the surgical procedure while the operative wound is open. However, this complication has been reported hours and even days after cataract extraction. When this occurs during the operation, the eye becomes firm and the patient may complain of severe pain if under local anesthesia. The wound opens, the iris prolapses, and if the lens has not been removed, it comes out spontaneously followed by vitreous, blood, and the rest of the intraocular contents. Sometimes it does not happen so violently and is preceded by decrease of the red reflex, followed by the appearance of an opaque mass in the vitreous space which grows progressively accompanied by obvious signs of increased intraocular pressure and other signs already described.

Intraoperative suprachoroidal hemorrhage was defined by three intraoperative criteria in a previous study conducted by Davison during extracapsular cataract surgery, a sense of progressively decreasing space in the anterior segment; a firm globe to tactile pressure; and the confirmation of a dark bulging suprachoroidal mass as observed at surgery by indirect ophthalmoscopy.[3]

It is important to clarify that the clinical picture, the behavior of the eye, and above all, the final consequences of this complication are totally different if the eye is undergoing planned extracapsular extraction with a limbal incision of 10 or 11 mm, or phacoemulsification with an incision of about 3 mm in length. The longer incision required by extracapsular techniques allows the intraocular contents to be expressed with relative ease should this complication occur. There is no time to close the wound with sutures. The situation is different when a phacoemulsification is being performed through a small self-sealing incision of 3 mm or less. During the procedure, the infusion maintains a stable anterior chamber and intraocular pressure. After removing the phaco handpiece, the internal lip of the self-sealing incision closes and allows the intraocular pressure to rise if the intraocular pressure increases. The increased intraocular pressure can tamponade the intraocular bleeding.

■ Management

One of the most perplexing and frustrating problems encountered during cataract surgery is shallowing of the anterior chamber with positive vitreous pressure. This condition may present at the outset of surgery or may occur at any stage during the procedure. By simply balloting the eye with the finger, the surgeon should be able to determine if the globe is firm. If so, the surgeon must suspect a suprachoroidal effusion or hemorrhage (Fig. 21–2). Careful inspection with the operating room microscope and a hand-held lens, or indirect ophthalmoscopy should confirm this problem. No stronger argument may be wagered for the use of a small self-sealing incision than in a case such as this.[9]

Another intraoperative cause for a firm globe is the aqueous or infusion deviation syn-

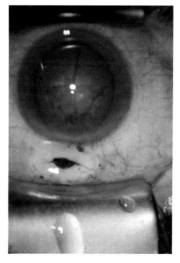

FIGURE 21–2. Intraoperative increase of intraocular pressure during phacoemulsification with iris prolapse through an ill-performed self-sealing incision.

drome. In these cases, surgery may be continued or temporarily delayed after administration of hyperosmotic agents. In extreme cases, a pars plana vitreous tap may be necessary.

When intraoperative suprachoroidal hemorrhage was suspected during ECCE or iris plane phacoemulsification, the recommendation was to stop the surgery, close the wound, and reoperate the next day when the anatomy had stabilized.

At present, the self-sealing anteriorly placed wound facilitates intraoperative containment even if digital pressure is applied. Digital massage has been used for years before the advent of such secure incisions.[10]

If an intraoperative suprachoroidal hemorrhage does occur, apply intermittent gentle digital massage with the index finger for a minimum of 10 minutes after filling the anterior chamber with a low cohesive high molecular weight viscoelastic material. This may allow completion of surgery as the suprachoroidal hemorrhage is contained. The viscoelastic material will act as an internal "balloon" with compensatory changes in vitreous volume. Remember that the only limiting factor to digital massage and waiting is the health of the retinal vasculature. If the central retinal artery becomes occluded, a vitreous tap might still be appropriate.

Controversy exists over the intraoperative management of this condition, but in limited cases the procedure may be completed. If at all questionable, however, surgery should be postponed and attention should be directed toward confirming the patency of the retinal vasculature.

It is difficult to predict the occurrence of this severe complication. Although risk factors exists, this condition has been reported in children and young adults in whom these alterations do not exist.

■ Tips and Pearls

1. Consider a patient as having a high risk for Acute Intraoperative Suprachoroidal Hemorrhage (AISH) in the presence of advanced age, glaucoma, increased intraocular pressure, increased axial length, and history of similar intraoperative complication in a previously operated eye.
2. The intraoperative presence of a shallow anterior chamber and a firm globe at tactile pressure should make you suspicious of the presence of this condition or of aqueous/infusion deviation syndrome.
3. AISH is confirmed at surgery with the use of the operating microscope and/or indirect ophthalmoscopy.
4. Fill the anterior chamber with low cohesive high molecular weight viscoelastic material and gently apply intermittent digital pressure with the index finger for a minimum of 10 minutes.
5. Confirm the patency of the retinal vasculature.
6. If at all questionable, surgery should be postponed.
7. There is less incidence of AISH during in-the-bag phacoemulsification surgery than the former techniques at iris-plane.
8. A small, self-sealing incision is mandatory in these high risk patients.

REFERENCES

1. Jaffe NS. Expulsive Hemorrhage. In: Welsh RC, Welsh J. (eds). The Second Report in Cataract Surgery. Miami: Educational Press; 1971;119–121.
2. Pau H. Der Ieitfaktor Bei Der Expulsiven Blitung. Klim Momats BL Augenheilild 1958;132:865–869.
3. Davison JA. Acute intraoperative suprachoroidal hemorrhage in capsular bag phacoemulsification. J Cataract Refract Surg 1993;19:534–537.
4. Manschot WA. The pathology of expulsive hemorrhage. Am J Ophthalmol 1955;40:15–24.
5. Hogan MJ, Zimmerman LE. Ophthalmic Pathology. Philadelphia: WB Saunders; 1962; 408.
6. Muller H. Expulsive hemorrhage. Trans Ophthalmol Soc UK 1959;79:621–634.
7. Speaker MG, Guerriero PN, Met JA, et al. A case-control study of risks factors for intraoperative suprachoroidal expulsive hemorrhage. Ophthalmology 1991;98:202–210.
8. Girard LJ. Expulsive hemorrhage during cataract surgery. Emergency treatment in five cases. In: Paton D (ed). Current Concepts in Cataract Surgery. Proceedings of the Third Biennial Cataract Congress. St. Louis: Mosby; 1974;612.
9. Nichamin LD. Prevention and management of complications. Ophthalmol Clin North Am 1995;8:523–538.
10. Osher MS. Emergency treatment of vitreous bulge and wound gaping complicating cataract surgery. Am J Ophthalmol 1957;44:409–411.

Index

Note: Figures and Tables are denoted by f and t respectively.

A

Acetaminophen, bleeding disorders, 167
Acute suprachoroidal hemorrhage, high myopia, 19
Anesthesia, bleeding disorders, 164–165
  cataract/glaucoma surgery, 83–84
  high hyperopia, 25–26, 25t
  high myopia, 15
  posterior polar developmental cataract, 23
  rock hard cataract, 115
  vitreoretinal surgery, 146
Anisometropia, high hyperopia, 26
Ankylosing spondylitis, uveitis, 72
Anterior capsulorhexis, posterior polar developmental cataract, 123
Anterior chamber, shallow, high hyperopia, 27–28
Anterior chamber intraocular lenses, uveitis, 69
Anterior cyclitic membrane, uveitis, 65–66, 66f
Anticoagulants, bleeding disorders, 161
Aphakia, piggyback IOL implantation, 10
Astigmatism, WTR, 38, 38f, 39t
Automated keratometry, corneal power determination, previous keratorefractive surgery, 6
Autorefractor/retinoscopy, intraoperative, previous keratorefractive surgery, 8
Axial length, intraocular lens power calculations, 1–3, 3t, 22
  triple procedure, 49

B

Behçet's disease, uveitis, 71–72, 71f-72f
Beehler pupil dilator, cataract/glaucoma surgery, 84, 92, 92f
  hyporeactive pupil, 58, 58f
Bleb, glaucoma, 76f-77f, 78, 79f, 80, 89f
Bleeding disorders, 161–168
  anesthesia, 164–165
  anticoagulants, 161
  examination, 162–164
  hemorrhagic diatheses, 162t
  incision, 165–166, 166f
  patient preparation, 164, 164t
  phacoemulsification technique, 166–167, 167f
  postoperative, 167–168
  surgical procedure, 164–167
Bullous keratopathy, 42f

C

Calculation method, corneal power determination, previous keratorefractive surgery, 4–5
Capsular contraction, subluxated cataract, 100–101
Capsular ring, glaucoma/pseudoexfoliation, 94–96, 95f
  subluxated cataract, 99–102
Capsulorhexis, glaucoma, 68
  intumescent cataract, 112–113
  pseudoexfoliation, 92–93

Capsulorhexis, glaucoma, *(continued)*
  rock hard cataract, 115–116
  uveitis, 68
Capsulotomy, subluxated cataract, 104, 104f
Cataract, etiology, 75
  Fuchs' corneal dystrophy, 42f
  post-RK, 8f
  post-RK and AK, 8f
  uveitis, 65–66, 66f
Cataract/glaucoma surgery
  anesthesia, 83–84
  complications, 87–88, 87f-88f
  postoperative, 87
  preoperative, 83
  surgical procedure, 83–87, 84f-86f
Children, 129–142
  cataract, associated ocular defects, 132
    classification, 131–132
    diagnosis, 130–131, 130f
    nonsurgical treatment defects, 132
    optical rehabilitation, 133, 133t
    postoperative care, 140–141
    preoperative evaluation, 132
    secondary IOL implantation, 140, 140f
    surgical procedure, 132, 134–140
      patient preparation, 134
      pupil dilation, 134
  eyes, anatomy, 120–130
Chop, chop, and stuff technique, rock hard cataract, 118, 118f
Choroidal detachments, cataract/glaucoma surgery, 87
Choroidal effusion, microphthalmia, 28
Choroidal hemorrhage, clinical manifestations, 175
  etiology, 173
  incidence, 173
  pathogenesis, 173–175
  surgical procedure, 175–176, 175f
Choroidal hemorrhage risk, 173–176
Chronic juvenile arthritis (CJA), uveitis, 68, 71
Chronic obstructive pulmonary disease (COPD), 157–160
  cough, 157
  oxygen therapy, 158
  patient positioning, 158–159, 158f-159f
  phacoemulsification, 159
Classification, preoperative, small pupil, 56, 56t

Clear corneal incision (CCI), bleeding disorders, 161
  Fuchs' corneal dystrophy, 43
  glaucoma, 76–77, 76f-77f, 78, 78f
  high astigmatism, 34–36, 34f-35f
  high hyperopia, 21, 27–28
  previous keratorefractive surgery, 8
  uveitis, 68
Clear corneal incision (CCI), subluxated cataract, 102, 102f, 104, 104f
Complications, cataract/glaucoma surgery, 87–88
  high hyperopia, 26
  high myopia, 19
  uveitis, 65–66
Congenital cataract, children, 132–133
Conjunctival limbal peritomy, cataract/glaucoma surgery, 84, 84f
Conjunctival repositioning, cataract/glaucoma surgery, 86, 86f
Conradi syndrome, 132
Continuous curvilinear capsulotomy, uveitis, 68
Cornea, peripheral, videokeratoscopic measurements, 51–52
Cornea guttata, 42f
Corneal power determination, previous keratorefractive surgery, 3–7
  automated keratometry, 6
  calculation method, 4–5
  corneal topography, 5–6
  manual keratometry, 6–7
  trial hard contact lens method, 5
Corneal protection, previous keratorefractive surgery, 8
Corneal topography, corneal power determination, previous keratorefractive surgery, 5–6
Cortical aspiration, glaucoma/pseudoexfoliation, 94
Crohn's disease, uveitis, 72
Cystoid macular edema, uveitis, 67, 70
  vitreoretinal surgery, 145, 149

D

Diabetic retinopathy, neovascularization of iris, 172
Diclofenac, uveitis, 67, 70
Digital massage, choroidal hemorrhage, 176
  glaucoma, 80

E

Effective lens position (ELP), 2
Endocapsular ring, subluxated cataract, 101, 101f
   vitreoretinal surgery, 148–149, 148f
Enlarged capsulotomy, subluxated cataract, 102, 103f
Epinucleus, rock hard cataract, 115
Epinucleus removal, posterior polar developmental cataract, 124f, 125–126
Extracapsular cataract extraction (ECCE), high myopia, complications, 19

F

Fixed pupil, 58–62
   evaluation, 56
   pupiloplasty, 60–62, 60f-62f
   stretch pupiloplasty, 58–60, 59f-60f
Foldable intraocular lenses, glaucoma, 78, 79f
   uveitis, 69
5-FU, cataract/glaucoma surgery, 87
   glaucoma, 80
Fuchs' corneal dystrophy, 41–47
   combined procedure vs. sequential surgery, 41–43, 43f
   examination, 41, 42f
   intraocular lens power calcuation, triple procedure, 45–56
   intraocular lens selection, 43
   perioperative evaluation, 41, 42f
   phacoemulsification with IOL, 43–45
   postoperative management, 46
   surgical procedure, 41–46
Fuchs' heterochromic cyclitis (FHC), uveitis, 70
Fulbiprofen, uveitis, 67

G

Galvanic cataract, 152f
Gimbel "phaco sweep," 93
Glaucoma, 75–81
   incision, 76–77, 76f-77f
   irrigation/aspiration, 78, 78f
   posterior synechias, 77
   postoperative, 80, 80f
   preoperative, 75–76
   pseudoexfoliation, 91–92
   small pupil, 77
Gonioscopy, glaucoma, 76

H

Heparin coated intraocular lenses, uveitis, 69
Herpes zoster, uveitis, 72
High astigmatism, 33–39
   astigmatic correction, 34–36
   intraocular lens power calculations, 33–34
   spherical correction, 33–34
   surgical procedure, 36–38, 37f-38f
High hyperopia, 21–31
   anesthesia, 25–26, 25t
   axial length measurement, 22
   challenges, 21–22
   complications, 26
   future, 30
   intraocular lens power calcuations, 21, 22–24, 23f-24f, 24t
   patient expectations, 26
   patient selection, 24–25
   piggyback IOL implantation, 22, 26, 27t, 28–29, 28f-29f
   postoperative refraction titration, 28
   shallow anterior chamber, 27–28
   surgical procedure, 26–27, 26t
High myopia, 13–19
   challenges, 14, 19
   defined, 13
   demographics, 13–14
   minus intraocular lens calculation, anterior chamber, 11
   postoperative, 18–19
      complications, 19
      refraction, 18–19
   preoperative evaluation, 14–15
      diagnosis, 14
      IOL caclulation, 14–15
      retina evaluation, 14
   surgical procedure, 15–18
      anesthesia, 15
      barrier preservation, 17, 17f-18f
      hydrodissection, 15
      incision, 15
      nucleus removal, 16, 17f
      pupillary dilation, 16–17
Hoffer Q T formula, high astigmatism, 33

Holladay 1 formula, high astigmatism, 33
  previous keratorefractive surgery, 2
Holladay 2 formula, high astigmatism, 33
  high hyperopia, 24, 26
  previous keratorefractive surgery, 3
Homocystinuria, 132
Hydrodelineation, posterior polar developmental cataract, 124
  rock hard cataract, 116
Hydrodissection, high myopia, 15
  posterior polar developmental cataract, 123–124
  pseudoexfoliation, 93
  rock hard cataract, 116
Hyphema, cataract/glaucoma surgery, 87
Hyporeactive pupil, Beehler pupil dilator, 58, 58f
  evaluation, 55–56
  iris hooks, 57, 57f
  Keuch pupil dilator, 58, 58f
  pharmacologic treatment, 56–57
  surgical techniques, 56–58
Hypotonous maculopathy, cataract/glaucoma surgery, 87, 87f

I

Immersion biometry, axial length measurement, 22
Inferior sphincterectomy, fixed pupil, 61–62, 62f–63f
Intracapsular cataract surgery (ICCE), high myopia, complications, 19
Intraocular lens insertion, cataract/glaucoma surgery, 85–86, 86f
  children, indications, 133t
  subluxated cataract, 106, 107f–108f
  vitreoretinal surgery, 148–149
Intraocular lens power calculations, 49–52
  axial length, 1–3, 3t, 22
  corneal power determination, previous keratorefractive surgery, 3–7
  Fuchs' corneal dystrophy, triple procedure, 45–56
  high astigmatism, 33–34
  high hyperopia, 21, 22–24, 23f-24f, 24t
  high myopia, 14–15
  limitations, 7
  piggyback IOL implantation, 9–11
  primary cataract surgery, 1–7

theoretical formulas, 1–3
  vitreoretinal surgery, 147
Intraoperative autorefractor/retinoscopy, previous keratorefractive surgery, 8
Intraoperative lens selection, uveitis, 66
Intraoperative suprachoroidal hemorrhage, criteria, 175
Intraoperative visualization, previous keratorefractive surgery, 8
Intumescent cataract, 111–114
  capsulorhexis, 111–114
    difficulties, 111–112
    phacoemulsification technique adaptation, 113
    strategy, 112–113
  challenges, 111
  white mature cataract, 113–114
IOL in-the-bag suture, 99
  zonular dehiscence, 107–109, 108f-109f
    surgical procedure, 108–109, 108f-109f
Iridectomy, cataract/glaucoma surgery, 86, 86f
  uveitis, 68
Iris, neovascularization, 169–172
Iris hooks, cataract/glaucoma surgery, 85
  hyporeactive pupil, 57, 57f
  uveitis, 67
Iris plane phacoemulsification, choroidal hemorrhage, 176
Iris protector ring, fixed pupil, 61, 61f-62f
Irrigation, subluxated cataract, 106, 107f

J

Juvenile rheumatoid arthritis (JRA), 132

K

Kammenn chopping technique, Fuchs' corneal dystrophy, 44–45, 45f
Kelman angled phaco needle, 148f
Keratometry, corneal power determination, previous keratorefractive surgery, 6–7
  postoperative, triple procedure, 49
Keratorefractive surgery, previous, 1–12
  corneal power determination, 3–7
  intraocular lens power calculation formulas limitations, 7
  piggyback IOL implantation, 3, 9–11
  postoperative evaluation, 8–9, 9f

postoperative refraction target selection, 7
preoperative evaluation, 7
surgical procedure, 8
Keuch pupil dilator, hyporeactive pupil, 58, 58f

L

Laser-assisted in-situ keratomileusis (LASIK), corneal power determination, 3–7
Lens cracking, glaucoma/pseudoexfoliation, 94
Lens fibers, rock hard cataract, 115
Limbal relaxing incision, high astigmatism, 34–36, 36f

M

Mackool technique, fixed pupil, 60–61, 60f-61f
Macular edema, neovascularization of iris, 172
Malignant glaucoma, cataract/glaucoma surgery, 88
Manual keratometry, corneal power determination, previous keratorefractive surgery, 6–7
Marfan syndrome, 132
subluxated cataract, 101–102, 102f
Mendez corneal ring, high astigmatism, 37, 37f
Microphthalmia, 132
Misdirection syndrome, cataract/glaucoma surgery, 88
Mitomycin C, cataract/glaucoma surgery, 87
Multifocal chorioretinitis, uveitis, 71–72
Multiple sphincterotomies, fixed pupil, 60, 60f
Mydriatics, hyporeactive pupil, 56

N

Neovascularization of iris, 169–172
etiology, 169
postoperative, 171–172
preoperative evaluation, 169–170
surgical procedure, 170–171, 170f-171f
Nucleus removal, high myopia, 16, 17f
posterior polar developmental cataract, 124–125, 124f

O

Ocular trauma, 151–156
diagnosis, 151–152, 152f
surgical procedure, 152–155

P

PAR visual system, high astigmatism, 38, 38f
Pars plana vitrectomy/lensectomy, uveitis, 68–69
Pars planitis, uveitis, 68, 71
Partial sphincterectomy, fixed pupil, 61, 62f
Pediatric IOL implantation, indications, 133t
Phaco snap procedure, bleeding disorders, 166–167, 167f
Phacoemulsification, chronic obstructive pulmonary disease (COPD), 159
glaucoma, 78, 78f
postoperative LASIK, long-term results, 9
postoperative PRK, long-term results, 9
postoperative RK, long-term results, 9
pseudoexfoliation, 93–94, 94f
subluxated cataract, 105–106, 106f
vitreoretinal surgery, 147–148
Photorefractive keratectomy (PRK), corneal power determination, 3–7
Piggyback IOL implantation, aphakia, 10
high hyperopia, 22, 26, 27t, 28–29, 28f-29f
previous keratorefractive surgery, 3, 9–11
IOL calcuations, 9–11
pseudophakia, 10–11
Polymethylmethacrylate (PMMA) lenses, Fuchs' corneal dystrophy, 43
subluxated cataract, 102
uveitis, 69
Posterior capsular opacification (PCO), intumescent cataract, 111
Posterior capsule opacification, high myopia, 19
Posterior capsulorhexis, posterior polar developmental cataract, 126
Posterior lenticonus, 130
Posterior polar developmental cataract, 121–128
challenges, 121
clinical study, 127–128
forms, 121, 122f
genetics, 122
incidence, 121

Posterior polar developmental cataract, (*continued*)
   pathogenesis, 122–123
   rupture predisposition, 123
   surgical procedure, 123–127
      anesthesia, 123
      anterior capsulorhexis, 123
      cortex removal, 126
      epinucleus removal, 125–126, 125f
      hydrodelineation, 124, 124f
      hydrodissection, 123–124
      incision, 123
      IOL fixation, 126–127, 126f
      nucleus removal, 124, 124f
      posterior capsulorhexis, 126
      rotation, 124
      viscoelastic material removal, 127
   symptoms, 121–122
Postoperative keratometry, triple procedure, 49
Postoperative phacoemulsification, previous RK, 9f
Postoperative refraction, high myopia, 18–19
Postoperative refraction target, selection, previous keratorefractive surgery, 7
Postoperative refraction titration, high hyperopia, 28
Postoperative retinal detachment, high myopia, 19
Prednisolone, glaucoma, 80
   uveitis, 70
Prednisone, uveitis, 67, 70
Preoperative classification, small pupil, 56, 56t
Preoperative refraction, piggyback IOL implantation, 10
   vs. axial length, piggyback IOL implantation, 9–10
Proxiphen, bleeding disorders, 167
Pseudoexfoliation, 91–96
   capsular ring, 94–96, 95f
   capsulorhexis, 92–93
   glaucoma, 91–92
   hydrodelineation, 93
   hydrodissection, 93
   phacoemulsification, 93–94, 94f
   small pupil, 92, 92f
Pseudophakia, piggyback IOL implantation, 10–11
   subluxated cataract, 101–102, 102f

Pupillary dilation, glaucoma, 7
   high myopia, 16–17
Pupiloplasty, fixed pupil, 60–62, 60f-62f

R

Radial keratotomy (RK), corneal power determination, 3–7
Refraction, preoperative, piggyback IOL implantation, 9–10
Refraction target, postoperative, selection, previous keratorefractive surgery, 7
Retina evaluation, high myopia, 14
Retinal detachment, postoperative, high myopia, 19
Rock hard cataract, 114–119
   anesthesia, 115
   capsulorhexis, 115–116
   chop, chop, and stuff technique, 118, 118f
   clinical study, 118t, 119
   difficulties, 114–115
   hydrodelineation, 116
   hydrodissection, 116
   incisional burns, 115
   lateral separation, 117–118, 117f-118f
   nuclear division, 116–117
   rotation, 116
   sculpting, 116
   step-by-step chop in situ, 117–118, 117f-118f
   surgical procedure, 115–119
   trench *vs.* crater, 116, 116f
   viscoelastics, 115
Rubeosis iridis, 169–172

S

Sanders-Retzlaff-Kraff/T (SRK/T) formula, triple procedure, 50
Sarcoidosis, uveitis, 70
Scleral tunnel incision, high astigmatism, 36
   previous keratorefractive surgery, 8
Sclerostomy, cataract/glaucoma surgery, 85, 85f
Silicone intraocular lenses, uveitis, 69
Slit lamp examination, Fuchs' corneal dystrophy, 42f
Small pupil, 55–64
   evaluation, 55–56
   glaucoma, 77

incidence, 55
postoperative, 62–64
preoperative, 55–56
pseudoexfoliation, 92, 92f
surgical procedure, 56–62
  fixed pupil, 58–62
  hyporeactive pupil, 56–58
SRK II formula, Fuchs' corneal dystrophy, 46
SRK/T formula, high astigmatism, 33
Step-by-step chop in situ, rock hard cataract, 117–118, 117f-118f
Stretch pupiloplasty, fixed pupil, 58–60, 59f-60f
Subluxated cataract, 99–110
  anterior lens capsule fixation, 103–107
    intraoperative lens selection, 103
    preoperative evaluation, 103
    small subluxation, 106–107
    surgical procedure, 103–106, 103f-106f
      capsulotomy, 104, 104f
        incision, 104, 104f
        IOL insertion, 106, 107f-108f
        irrigation/aspiration, 106, 107f
        phacoemulsification, 105, 106f
        suturing, 104–105, 104f-106f
  capsular ring, 99–102
    implantation, 100, 100f
    indications, 100–102, 101f-103f
  IOL in-the-bag suture, 107–109, 108f-109f
Superior sector iridectomy, fixed pupil, 62, 63f
Surprofen, uveitis, 67
Synechias, posterior, glaucoma, 77
Syphilis, uveitis, 70–71

T

Theoretical formulas, intraocular lens power calculations, 1–3
  vs. empirical formulas, 26
Toxoplasmosis, uveitis, 72
Trabeculectomy flap, cataract/glaucoma surgery, 84, 84f
Trial hard contact lens method, corneal power determination, previous keratorefractive surgery, 5
Triamcinolone, uveitis, 67
Triple procedure, Fuchs' corneal dystrophy, 41–43, 43f
  glaucoma/pseudoexfoliation, 91

intraocular lens power calculations, 49–52
refractive results, 49–50, 50t

U

Ultrasound axiometers, axial length measurement, 22
Uveitis, 65–72
  ankylosing spondylitis, 72
  anterior, 72
  Behçet's disease, 71–72, 71f-72f
  challenges, 65
  chronic juvenile arthritis (CJA), 68, 71
  complications, 65–66, 70
  Crohn's disease, 72
  Fuchs' heterochromic cyclitis (FHC), 70
  herpes zoster, 72
  intraoperative lens selection, 66
  multifocal chorioretinitis, 71–72
  ocular inflammation control, 65
  pars planitis, 68, 71
  patient preparation, 67
  postoperative inflammation, 66
  postoperative treatment, 69–70
  preoperative inflammation, 67
  sarcoidosis, 70
  surgical technique, 67–69
    combined cataract-vitrectomy, 68–69
    intraocular lenses, 69
    phacoemulsification, 68
  syphilis, 70–71
  toxoplasmosis, 72
  visual prognosis, 65
  Vogt-Koyanagi-Harada, 71–72

V

Videokeratoscopic measurements, peripheral cornea, 51–52
Vitrectomy, uveitis, 68
Vitreoretinal surgery, 145–149
  anesthesia, 146
  examination, 146
  history, 145–146
  intraocular lens power calculations, 147
  intraocular lens selection, 146–147
  intraoperative, 147
  postoperative, 149
  preoperative, 145–147

Vitreoretinal surgery, *(continued)*
  surgical procedure, 146–149
Vitreous prolapse, subluxated cataract, 101, 101f
Vogt-Koyanagi-Harada, uveitis, 71–72

W

White mature cataract, 113–114
Wilson disease, 132

Wound leaks, cataract/glaucoma surgery, 87
WTR astigmatism, 38, 38f, 39t

Z

Zonular dialysis, ocular trauma, 153f-154f
Zonular disinsertion, subluxated cataract, 101, 101f
Zonules, glaucoma/pseudoexfoliation, 93
  subluxated cataract, 99